Reviews

"This very personalised guide-book to th to chronic back pain is both comprehens approach.

As a doctor I believe it is medically safe and sound as a valuable resource to those who have failed to benefit from the panoply of treatments for this disabling condition.

Ironically, while reading this book I suffered from several weeks of an unaccustomed stiff lower back, and I was able to appreciate the relevance of this publication and the great insights with which it has been written."

Dr David Brownridge
Retired General Practitioner, Fellow of the British Medical
Association & Chairman of the Worcestershire and
Herefordshire division of the BMA

"This is an excellent read offering very sound and sensible advise to all 'back pain' sufferers.

The way Peter has written this book and the positive approach to his long term management is a credit to him and could be applied to many other medical conditions which involve immobility and pain.

As Peter says: 'Take ownership of your problems do not abdicate health care to anyone, work in partnership and take action to help yourself."

Magdeline Coomber
Retired Nurse teacher and specialist nurse in
Gastroenterology and Diabetes

"This book is brilliant, it gives lots of practical and useful information that you just won't find anywhere else. It is inspirational, it has even got me doing some of the exercises and they really do make a difference."

Heidi Barnsley IIHHT
Advanced Sport Therapist

"Peter's book is inspirational, motivating, hopeful and reassuring. It encourages self-control, choice and independence. He is mindful of the relationship between conventional medicine and complementary therapies and his recommendations are not whacky off-the-wall ideas but practical and achievable approaches. I am sure this book will help many to overcome pain and immobility and the associated distress and loss of dignity. Peter is proof that with practice and determination, people can have the power within them to change predicted outcomes.

Working as a nurse for nearly 40 years, I have seen many colleagues impacted by back injury, sometimes terminating careers early, often debilitated for lengths of time or seemingly permanently. If this book goes some way to improving health and well-being and self-worth, then it is worth every moment invested in reading it."

Nicky West RGN, DN, Dip Pall Care, Cert MMt
Nurse & Hospice CEO

"As a back pain sufferer of many years standing, I have found that, like Peter, there is no magic bullet. You have got to keep moving, keep trying different things and work through the pain – this book explains how and shows there is a way forward."

"Peter's tips, methods, procedures and above all practical advice give us fellow sufferers more ideas and thoughts on how to cope and critically how to live an active, positive life. "

Michael Kay
Back pain sufferer

"This book kept me on my toes at a time when depression was kicking in due to the inability to work and when everything was an immense effort. The action points helped to make me more positive and responsible

I now think about how I sit, walk and do everyday tasks and also I'm able to incorporate my exercises into my daily routine.
All the advice in this book is very valuable and is a must for anyone with any back problems, it has the ability to make you want to get up and restart your life."

Denise Brown
Back pain sufferer

"Peter Johnson's book is highly informative and provides detailed, practical advice to remedy back pain. He has explored and developed strategies for managing every aspect of daily life and given hope to those who live with this debilitating condition."

Jackie Lush
Back pain sufferer

"This book represents a victory for common sense and personal discipline to overcome back pain, that is achievable by anyone with little determination. Peter comes to the subject from a deeply personal perspective, he carefully weighs up various therapies and gives his considered advice in practical and achievable steps. The book confronts the difficulties head-on with compassion and clear thinking, it is an excellent read."

Mr R L J Douglas-Bate

"At last a book that speaks common sense! Written by someone who's walked the path of back pain and was determined to get back literally on his feet. This book is full of great practical advice.

My personal experience was being told to 'rest up' until being seen by a specialist nine months later to be told not only was that the worst advice but it's actually exacerbated my condition. This book puts the ownership of the issue firmly back (!) into the readers hands, making small adjustments to reduce pain, increase comfort and, of course, mobility.

If you're serious about not being held back, this book is for you."

Sallie Bate
Back pain sufferer

*"**What better way to cure your back problems, than to learn from someone who has done it.** 80% of people will suffer from a back problem at some point in their lives. Be it a niggle or outright agony, all back pain has a debilitating effect on life, effecting drive, desire and confidence. While the medical route can help, there is also a natural path. In "I beat back pain so can you" Peter Johnson provides an honest, holistic approach to curing back problems. It looks at fear, exercise, work, diet and more in a practical, no-hype manner. It's a must read if you genuinely want to beat back pain in a natural way. What better way to cure your back problems, than to learn from someone who has done it."*

Neil Fellowes
Helping people objectively see what works for their health
www.totalwellness.club

"One of the most easily understood and informative books on back pain I have ever read. This book sets out ways in which you can deal with the problems and ensure that you don't suffer in the same way in the future. There are simple steps I use in my everyday life which seem common sense now but needed to be there is black and white before I realised the difference they could make."

Lee Gough
Back pain sufferer

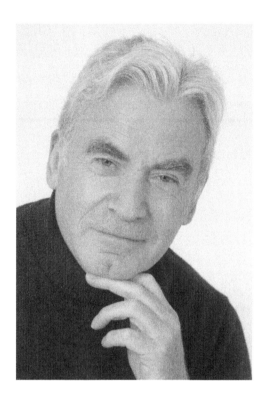

Peter Johnson

Former Back Pain Sufferer

Peter Johnson is a businessperson who suffered a major back problem at the height of his career. Determined to get better, without surgery or drugs, he applied his business-like approach to research, trial and regain full pain-free mobility. He runs his own business consultancy, is highly qualified, and became the 1st person in the world accredited in one of his specialist fields. His pragmatism is evident in his work, speaking and writing.

www.TheBackChampion.com

I Beat Back Pain

So Can You

Cure Back Pain
Without Surgery Or Drugs

Peter Johnson

www.TheBackChampion.com

Copyright

Formerly titled: *Wave Goodbye to Back Pain*

For all sufferers and people wishing to avoid back pain
– there is a way forward.

Preface

We all know someone who is suffering from back pain and most of us have experienced it personally. In some cases, the bouts of pain may be occasional but in many it is a permanent agony that can blight a person's life totally. Because it is so prevalent many books have been written on the subject.

This book is different. It is not written by a medical specialist or a professional in related fields, nor does it contain impenetrable technical language or propose expensive technical remedies. The author is a person who, in the prime of an active life, found his world collapsing around him. He was even warned that he could lose the capacity to walk. This is his personal story of how, through sheer determination, hard work and exercise, as well as perseverance in changing all aspects of his way of living, he fought his way back to a full and healthy life. His book is not just an example of what can be done but is full of practical, simple and often obvious ways in which you can do the same and banish back pain.

Dame Margaret J Anstee DCMG
Former Under-Secretary General
United Nations

Disclaimer

Peter Johnson is neither a medical practitioner or medically trained. The content of this book is offered in good faith based on research and action undertaken by him to remedy his lower back pain. He cannot, nor will not, guarantee that the contents of this publication will work for you and accepts no liability for any results you achieve.

Always consult a qualified medical practitioner. Act responsibly and if excessive pain or strain is experienced in attempting any of the actions explained in this book or if anyone is under medical supervision it is recommended to follow the advice of their doctor, professional medical advisor or physiotherapist, particularly before undertaking any exercises.

Contents

Author's Story

A few years ago I had a major back problem that robbed me of the ability to walk. My life was in turmoil and I went from a person with high personal drive and capability to a person who was struggling to get by. I did get by, and then got better and I thought that was normal and the end of the story. But for most people is it? I have sadly found out that for many this is just the beginning of a life full of limitations.

Not so long ago I was sharing my story with a room of 120 highly motivated people – suddenly realising that what I had achieved was not so ordinary after all and worth sharing.

I really did have a true 'ahh ha moment'. And this is why I was encouraged to write this book.

In a room on a grey November day I shared only a fraction of my story of how I had regained my life and mobility after a serious back problem – I was shocked by the reaction in the room as so many people came up to me and said how amazing it was and I must write down what I had done.

They had friends and family and even some people in the room were suffering with back pain – they wanted to know what I had done – how I had cured my back pain. They wanted to know so they could help the people they care about, help them regain their lives too. A few days later the gentleman who was running the weekend workshop sent out a letter saying 'Peter's story brought a tear to my eye'.

I should say that the workshop was nothing to do with back pain or alternative therapies. It was on strategies for developing successful businesses, so no link what so ever – but life is odd like that isn't it?

So I decided to reveal what I did and what I still do to keep free from pain and able to lead an active, and dare I say 'normal' life.

If I start at the beginning I have to wind the clock back many years. I was a very fit and capable sports person in my school days and undertook a vast range of sports. All very competitively and all to a high standard. These were the days when you just got on and played the game, warming up was not always something you did. Pre and post activity stretching was also not usual like it is today. We called getting fit and prepared, 'training', unlike sports people today who call it 'work'. Rehydration was a word that meant nothing. We had a post event drink and if we were thirsty during an event it was highly unusual to get anything. On the rugby field at half time we had a slice of orange. How times have changed, both on and off the sports field.

Many years ago I had a serious lower back pain problem and ended up in bed for weeks. This was followed by a week in hospital in traction. I was refused surgery and then encased in plaster from waist to neck. Not fun I can assure you, especially during a hot summer!

Months later I started to go back to work part time. I could not drive and everything was a real effort. I felt wretched but my wife and family were wonderful taking the strain of everyday life and driving me if I needed to go anywhere.

My back eventually started to mend and after several months I was able to hobble around. I had lost weight and had constant pain down my legs – a pain that was to remain for the next 5 years. It took a long time to start to return to a normal life. I had a further major relapse some years later and avoided surgery a second time – again a very debilitating time and one that took a long time to recover from.

After my wife became ill, and whilst caring for her I unknowingly seriously damaged my back. Sadly she died and it was shortly after this that I had a major problem. Suddenly my whole life had fallen apart.

I had a great job with a large organisation and the future looked very rosy. My employers were very understanding but I knew that I was in a bad way. What to do?

My medical general practitioners were brilliant and did all that they could to help me, but ultimately the diagnosis was not good. The X-rays and subsequent MRI scans showed that the lower part of my back was massively damaged and I had a series of 'slipped discs'. The pain was monumental, the disabling effect was ridiculous – I could do so little when I was used to doing so much – work was not even on my radar, just surviving was my only aim.

I had gone from being a fully achieving sort of person to someone who struggled to get out of a chair – I mean really struggled.

To give you a little insight into what it meant for me, it was a truly terrifying experience to try and stand up from a chair. You know it is going to hurt; you brace yourself and still cannot believe the pain as it hits your whole body. People think it is just your back – it is not, it affects your whole body. You cannot breath properly, your body is in tension and this white heat of pain burns its way into you as you even try and move a fraction. Sometimes it is just enough to grovel to the floor and crawl. Each movement sending a shockwave of pain through you. The cold sweat starts, the groaning helps and if no one else is about you can curse (eventually you don't care and curse anyway). Then the 15 minutes journey to the kitchen or the toilet starts.

I remember one day when I was getting my dinner it took two journeys and an hour to peel one carrot. Yes, one carrot. I earned my dinner that day! I could have asked a friend to call in and help. I could have asked my parents but I needed my space and more importantly I needed to try and keep some dignity.

Suddenly my life was shattered. I had gone from being a fully able and functioning adult who did a wide variety of things to someone for whom the simplest task was a major challenge.

I developed a phrase which helped me get some focus: The 'Pain maybe inevitable, the suffering is optional.'

When I think back, a simple hug from a loved one was a missed pleasure because of the physical pain that it brought. The thought of friends children rushing up to give me a hug.... and then stopping knowing that I 'was different', that I could not play rough and tumble with them on the floor. So painful in a very different way.

The list of what I could not do went on....

- Putting a log on the fire
- Nipping out to get that take-out for a night in watching a film
- Popping down the pub to see friends
- Out for a round of golf
- To the sports game with friends and family
- The missed dinner invitations
- The missed parties
- Not being able to cook dinner for friends and families
- The acceptance by friends and family that they won't get that birthday card or present

And still the list went on...

The doctors were great but there was little that could be done, or so it seemed, unless I started to consider surgery.

Surgery was the obvious next step and this works for some but often it is not always the success it is made out to be. Many people who have surgery have relapses, especially with complex cases. This is not the route I wanted – it *may* have worked, but *may* was not good enough.

I tried a range of alternative therapies and to this day I respect the physiotherapist who said 'sorry Peter I am out of my range here, this is just too bad'. He knew me well from past episodes, had an excellent reputation and had vast experience. I heard his words and thanked him for his honesty but inside the fear was terrible.

I tried a recommended top chiropractor who after a series of sessions and looking at some X-rays said that it was unlikely I would ever walk properly again. This was not *me* he was talking about my head screamed, it's that other ashen looking guy bent and twisted in pain who just happens to wear the same clothes as me that I saw in his full length mirror.

I did huge amounts of research and eventually found a brilliant Neurosurgeon. I was still trying to avoid surgery.

He indicated that with the problems I had there was no guarantee of success and any failure was not good news at all. My chances he said were low. Surprisingly, he was very forthright with his view on surgery. He felt that in the vast majority of cases surgery is the incorrect treatment.

He also shook me cold when he said that if I carry on living life the way I did I would probably be in a wheel chair by the time I was 50. I left his consulting rooms in a daze and realised that the person all of these specialists talked about was in fact me. This journey was mine. It was up to me, and me alone to make the decision – I just knew I had to do something.

It was after much thought, research, challenge and digging deep I developed my way of getting better. The journey I developed required many excellent people, including the Neurosurgeon (no surgery though), a lot of trial and error, even more trial and pain. A lot of time researching a broad range of topics that I did not even know existed. A huge amount of cash and a faith that I would be able to walk again. That I would still be walking beyond 50 and the full intention of enjoying life.

The journey I undertook has meant that I reclaimed my mobility, I eventually got rid of the chronic back pain and my life started to return to normal – well as normal as it could be after the death of my wife. Now I could start to grieve and rebuild my life. I have developed a way of managing my back, it is no longer an issue for me and few people now ask 'how is your back?' which was always the first question anyone would say. I became 'Hi-Peter-how's-your-back' – yes, it was lovely that people cared and were concerned and helpful but it was almost as if I had lost my own identity.

I identified a whole range of things that I did to regain my life, my mobility, my future – a full and good life after 'the back'. These are shared in this book.

Just for clarification I confirm I take no medication and I have had no surgery. I have avoided injections in my back. I use no 'appliances' and my home looks normal and is not full of aids and devices. I drive a normal car (well in fact I don't – I love sports cars and had a classic 1960s MG for a while once I was better, a few other low fast cars too.) I ride a standard bicycle, everything is 'normal' including my enthusiasm for each new day.

I am not a medical person – just someone who was determined to get better and whilst I cannot guarantee everything will work for everyone what I share are the exact same things that have worked for me.

It has taken many years to prove these things work and I now know that they work for me. I also know that whilst I cannot guarantee they will work for everyone I am certain that there are things that I have shared that will make a significant difference. The only thing that you need is the commitment to use them. I know my life was worth the effort – I am sure yours is too.

Someone I know shared this extract from a book with me after I was better and it resonated with me. It may resonate with you too:

> *"To see illness as symbolic and to accept complete responsibility for them will be most hard for those who hide behind their physical condition, and use their illness and disability as a 'crutch; to help them through life (no pun intended). For if I am sick and ill, then I can expect sympathy, I can be excused from dealing with the travails that an active life can bring me. I can demand that society supports me... the list goes on. There can be advantages as well as disadvantages in being ill. In many instances illness and disability can be a very useful tool in avoiding facing up to life; can be a ready-made excuse for not partaking fully in life."*

'Are we there yet?' – Dennis D Hunt

The only person in your way is probably yourself, I was determined to get out of my own way and get better.

I was also determined never to be termed 'disabled'. There are many deserving cases where people do have no choice and I believe they should have respect and support. I therefore made a choice that I would never act like someone who was disabled. I have never used parking places for people who need them, even if it meant getting wet on a rainy day. With hindsight I believe this attitude really did help my recovery as I forced myself to do things that I could so easily have made easier.

I trialled a whole series of various therapies. Some were certainly not for me and some were lovely. Some seemed to do some good. Some did cause a problem and some were just pleasant at the time. It took a lot of trial, money and at times painful error to find what worked for me and I have shared these thoughts in the chapter on therapies.

The one thing I can certainly say is there is no instant cure for lower back pain, middle back pain or any other back pain.

I bought and tried many appliances and pieces of equipment in an attempt to make life easier. I found most of them to be a waste of money and soon realised that I just had to get on with things. These were things that didn't work. Also because they were 'specialist' they were very expensive, and as I found out, most were useless. I even bought things that caused more problems!

Importantly I realised at an early stage that they were making me dependent upon them. My home was starting to look less 'homely'. I had to move things so other people could sit down and it then struck me the way I was adapting everything. I made a decision to start to clear these things out of my home, and out of my life.

I will admit that I have purchased a top quality office chair and my desk, which I got from IKEA, does have legs that are adjustable for height. That is about it, but I do spend significant hours working at my desk so believe it is well justified.

When I was first ill I had a lovely executive car, which was very comfortable to drive. Once I left corporate life I have had a series of sports and sporty cars including a 1960s Classic MG sports car. None have been a problem and none have had any adjustments, as I was keen to make sure that life was normal.

After I got back on my feet my life started to return to some sort of normality but I still had this concern that at any moment I would have a major relapse. It was always there...

- Should I go on holiday?
- Could I manage a long flight?
- What if I had a problem when I was walking by myself?
- What if I did something stupid?
- What if.....?

- What if....?
- What if.... This was still no way to live.

I had to stop these questions and just get on with life.

One day I was asked to do something that made me dig deep into myself. I was asked to lead a group of people on a charity trek to the base camp of the highest mountain in Tibet – wow!! These people had never known me with a back problem and had only ever seen me as a fit man – there was no agenda, only my internal one.

But then the 'what ifs' started thick and fast.

You can imagine the concerns I had after what you have learnt about my problem.

- What if I had a problem on the mountain?
- What if I let these people down?
- What if I couldn't get up one morning?
- What if I slowed everyone down?
- What if……

Anyway to cut a long story short I went to Tibet with only 6 weeks preparation and intensive training – I was so proud of the people who had raised huge amounts of money and achieved the pinnacle of this adventure.

Not everyone reached the base camp for various reasons but everyone was a major achiever. They had conquered the mountain in one way or another but more importantly they had all achieved far more than they had ever done in the past. We trekked to 16,000 feet in one of the remotest parts of the world. And yes, I had done it too, the 'what ifs?' started to fade away.

I wondered if this was a one off? That was put to the test soon enough as my next challenge was to climb what are called 'The 3-peaks'. This is where we climb to the top of the highest mountains in England, Scotland and Wales – namely Scarfell Pike, Ben Nevis and Snowdon – in a weekend. A well known and tough challenge – I did that too.

The tears of achievement that we all shed on those days were a far cry from those that I had shed when wracked in pain not so long before; fearing that my active life was over. I can cross country ski – that means skiing uphill as well as downhill – and when people ask 'why?' I just say 'because I can!' knowing once I just couldn't. I hill walk, swim, cycle and I also collapse in front of the TV with a beer.

I have since undertaken some other adventures too and my main question now is to establish if it will fit into my busy diary – not if my back will allow me to do it. Fantastic!

The results I have created have been life changing. I went from someone who had an hour and half of white knuckle agony to get up in the morning to get to the bathroom and dressed. To get up to a day of struggling in pain. I now spring out of bed eager for the day ahead.

I run my own business whereas I could not even think _to_ work, let alone _of_ work. I can entertain friends and happily cook a full meal whereas before a very simple dinner for one was a major challenge.

I still sometimes stop and think when I make a cup of tea, just what a challenge it once was.

As I said non-judgementally earlier – "The only person in your way is probably yourself." **Now step aside and make way for the real you!**

I wish you well.

Introduction

Of all of the problems that can cause pain and immobility there are few worse than severe back pain. The statistics are frightening and give some idea of the suffering that this ailment causes.

Just for the UK and USA:

> It is estimated that back pain affects 80% of people at some point during their lives in the industrialised world, and roughly 40% of all workplace absences have been due to back pain.

In the USA

- About 31 million Americans are affected by lower back pain.
- Back pain is the second most common reason for visiting a doctor.
- 50% of the Americans who are working suffer from back pain each year.
- Approximately $50 billion is being spent on back pain by Americans each year.

In the UK

- Nearly 5 million working days are lost as a result of back pain each year. This means that on any one day 1% of the working population are on sick leave due to a back problem.
- Back pain is the second most common reason for visiting a doctor.
- The NHS spends more than £1 billion each year on back pain related costs. A further £600million is spent in the private healthcare sector. A further £600million is the estimated cost to employers.

Sources: Various

Introduction

It is understandable why some people never get better and live a life of making do and struggling each and every day. It is understandable why the medical profession is so besieged with patients visiting with their problems. It is also sadly understandable that there is inadequate time in most consulting rooms and doctors surgeries for there to be a full and comprehensive diagnosis that most practitioners would like to provide.

The genesis of this book was a two-day business programme that I attended totally unrelated to health issues. It was one of those serendipitous moments that happen every now and then! Following a conversation at lunchtime with someone I had met earlier in the day I was encouraged to share with the 120 people in the room what became an 'ah ha' moment at the end of the first day.

I said little more than:

> Following the death of my wife, at too early an age, whilst looking after her I had created a reoccurrence of my back problems. In the very early stages of this back problem I was barely able to move, in extreme pain and unable to work. Quickly I knew I had a big problem – a problem much worse than I had had before. I needed to accept responsibility for getting better and deal with it quickly so I could resume a normal life. It became clear, and I was advised that if I continued to carry on the way I was, I risked being unable to ever walk properly again and probably be in a wheel chair at 50. I also mentioned that to prove to myself that I had finally regained normality I took a group of people to the base camp of the highest mountain in Tibet.

That was my brief story – the longer version can be found at the start of this book.

Introduction

The impact was amazing – over the following few hours at least 75% of the people in the room came and spoke to me telling stories of their back problems, those of friends and family who were in pain and not getting better, or living lives well below their potential. Lives, from the stories that could, it seemed, be much better. I was told I must write a book about my story – this is that book.

I cannot guarantee what works for me will work for you. I can only share what I did, and do to live an active life, when there was the probability I would be inactive. My back pain was in my lower back although this book is written with back pain sufferers generally in mind.

It has taken longer than I had imagined to complete. I needed to consider the journey I had taken, and what I had done, as much is now a part of my normal life.

It is seldom there is one single thing that makes the difference.

You can make a lot of difference with a collection of small individual things, as I have discovered from the research I have undertaken. So what I'm taking you through is the whole journey of everything I put in place. Some are minute things but if you put those small grains on the scales, each grain adds weight. Eventually it tips from being a person with a bad back to a person who lives a great life.

Your journey can start as soon as you read the first page.

Do be responsible and if in any doubt seek medical advice.

I wish you well.

Introduction

How to use this book

It was mentioned in the introduction there is unlikely to be just one area of this book, or any book, that makes *the* difference. It will be a compounding of a range of things across the whole book.

The chapters have been placed in an order that I believe works, but it is in no way a strict reading order and you may well want to dip into later chapters at an early stage, especially if you see a heading that catches your eye. If this works for you that is great so go ahead. I do encourage you to read all the chapters though.

At the end of each chapter there are a few action points to consider and they are written in a way to encourage you take action. They are not exhaustive summaries of the chapter. There will be many more actions that you should consider within each chapter – so do read through – the action points are just a start.

Crucially there is no point in reading things and not taking action – action is the key to getting better.

Take small steps first and build on them. Add in steps from differing areas too. They all add up.

The final tips I will give are:

- Have a pen and book of blank paper, large diary or a ring binder and some clean paper available as soon as you start reading so you can make notes. Use this as the place where you keep a history of how things are developing.

- Make notes! And date them.

How to use this book

- When you start to do something chart what you do and the impact it has over the coming days and weeks.

- If you feel what is suggested will cause excess pain and deterioration in your condition don't do it.

- Involve your medical practitioner.

- Take one small action as soon as you can so you start on your journey....then you will be ready for the next step.

Chapter 1

Combating the fear of back pain

Why understanding this is so important

One of the biggest challenges about dealing with back problems is the fear that both the pain and the lack of mobility have on a person's life. This fear in itself is enough to stop many people from starting to reclaim a more active and less painful life.

A key aspect of this book will be to encourage you to take action so that you can reclaim much of the mobility that you have lost. It is also aimed at helping you reduce the level of pain that you are suffering so that you can move forward and start to feel the relief and progress of reclaiming one's life.

One of the biggest challenges is realising that there is a future beyond the debilitating effects of back pain and where you are at the moment.

There are a few back-related problems that are chronic and will not allow people to regain the mobility and the pain free life that they had before. However, many people end up caught in the belief that now that they have back pain and back problems it is a permanent feature of their life. They just give up the challenge to get better, assuming it is a lost cause and there is little hope. This is not the case.

Additionally, the fear that many people have is that they will need to take painkillers and other medication for the long term just to maintain some element of normality in their life. This is also not the case.

Chapter 1 – Combating the fear of back pain

Back pain can be fought by adopting a significant range of self-treatment methods that will be explained in this book. These are easy to incorporate into a 'normal' lifestyle. They are part of regaining the life style you had before.

The fear in itself will be a restricting factor so you need to combat this aspect and what you are going through. The fear can hold you back and you will be frightened of taking any steps that will cause you additional discomfort. It is totally understandable that there will be fear and concern but do not let this stop you taking action.

There is also the fear of the effect that your restriction will have on relationships, family life, socialising, any sport you do, normal everyday activities and of course work. This is completely normal and understandable.

One of the biggest problems with people getting better from their back pain is combating the fear and just taking action. You will be taken through everything you need to know. Indeed, I will be sharing everything that has formed the integrated parts of what I did to regain mobility and a pain free life.

It is worth bearing in mind that those close to you may also be afraid of the dramatic change they have seen in you. The lack of mobility, the pain and the way it has impacted on their lives too. Whilst being mindful of this you must not dwell on it and add other stresses and strains on top of your own.

If those who are close see you are taking a proactive approach and really trying to get mobile and better this will reassure them too.

It may seem counter intuitive to risk doing anything that could seem to play to the pain but this is one of the main reasons why so many people don't do anything – because of the fear.

Their focus is on fear. Your focus will be on getting on with your life.

ACTION

- What are you focusing on right now – is it fear or something positive?

- If you fear the way you feel, decide to take control.

- Start right now to do something that will give you hope.

- Commit to reading this book and taking action with the points raised.

Chapter 1 – Combating the fear of back pain

Chapter 2

How to deal with relapses

Before we go any further it is important to address the area of relapses. You may have none, which is fantastic, but there is the possibility you will. Do not worry.

One of the devastating parts of having a serious back problem is that periodically you may well have relapses. There are two ways of looking at these:

- Firstly, very negatively, as it feels as if all your hard work has been wasted for no result at all.
- Or secondly, with a dramatically different approach and think of them as small challenges on the road to recovery.

The very fact that we are having periodic relapses means that we are challenging ourselves and our bodies to improve. A key part about a speedy recovery is to take any relapse in your stride.

Yes, you may want to feel sorry for yourself for a while but do not let this stop you for any length of time. It is really important that you continue with your self-treatment as soon as possible. You may have to go back to undertaking much more limited tasks and fewer repetitions in any type of exercises that you are undertaking. This will be explained later in this book. Do not see this as a failure – I am certain that your speed of recovery will be much quicker if you keep going. Treat these as minor hiccups with the intention of returning to the level of performance that you had reached before. Critically, measure the change that you have had due to the relapse in your normal daily recordings – this is all outlined in chapter 13 because it will give you:

- A clear insight into how far you have regressed (albeit on a temporary basis).
- It will also give you a good history on how your back is performing.
- It will also give you a very clear view whether any activity you are undertaking is having a detrimental effect on the health of your back.
- It is a great time to consider what you have done differently that may cause you a problem.

Examples may include that you have started to sit in your own 'comfortable' chair again. Or you have failed to do your exercise regime for the last few days. Or maybe you have done something too strenuous, which with hindsight was too much. Do think things through, equally importantly though don't over analyse the situation and talk yourself down. Move on.

I had a number of relapses. For some it was clear what I did that caused the problem. For others I have no idea of the reason. Once I got used to this I did not over analyse and moved forward again.

No matter what state you have reached both mentally or physically **I cannot recommend strongly enough for you to continue or start your back care regime today.** Failure to do so will mean all of the work that you have put in so far will be wasted. The strength that you have started to build will be lost within a matter of days if you don't continue with your exercises. The disappointment will continue unless you carry on doing something to move yourself forward. As I mentioned earlier, any relapse really should be viewed as a small stumbling point on the journey to greater health. If you have been undertaking all aspects recommended within this book you will be positioning yourself for a more mobile and less painful life.

A potential problem of any relapse is that it makes us lose faith in what we are doing. It makes one wonder if what we are doing is causing more pain. One of the biggest setbacks is the sheer effort of having to get going and it makes us feel as if we are starting all over again. The reality is the opposite. What it frequently indicates is that we are getting much better and it is the extra effort that we have made that is part of the healing process.

Just think what can happen if you have been unfit and then decide to do some serious exercise. For example, we go on a very long walk having not walked for a long time, or go to the gym after a long lazy holiday. After such events it is not unusual to ache or feel very stiff – any relapse is, in many ways, no different.

Because we have been feeling much better we may have forgotten and lifted that heavy item not realising just how heavy it was, or twisted suddenly to do something, or not picked something up as we know we should have. All of these things cause relapses, and often we can pinpoint what it was. Often we cannot though and this makes us concerned about what it actually was.

We have all spoken to people we know who have never had a back problem and then out of the blue they have a problem. Completely unexpected – so don't get concerned. No matter how fit and well anyone is, back problems happen. So treat any future problem, just as a 'one off' and get on with things. Don't assume that your main back problem has come back. By adopting many of the things explained in this book there is no reason why you cannot live a life where a back problem is a distant memory. And any future problem you treat as if it were your first. Easy to say, very difficult to do – but well worth the effort.

The reality is if you adopt what this book covers, any future problem you encounter you will be able to deal with quickly. Far quicker than anyone who does not know this material.

Also, one of the problems with relapses is that they can niggle and we start to get tired as we cannot sleep as well. We worry about the impact this is having on our lives and it all starts to be a downward spiral – you can stop this by taking ownership of the problem and deciding to do something about it.....straight away.

You will meet many people who are happy to tell you how bad things are but they are not prepared to do anything to sort things out. You have, at your fingertips, all you need to know to take charge, to take control of the situation. The choice is always yours.

Also look under the chapter 10 which is on 'stress' and you will realise that some of the things that can stop you getting back to good health quickly will be stress related. The more you worry, the greater the stress you inflict on yourself and the slower it will be to move forward!

Minor relapses

I'll deal with the easiest ones first. Most adults in the western world have a back problem at some time in their adult life – this is a statement of fact. If you meet someone with a back problem it may be they've had a twinge, they have done something daft, like lifting something too heavy or spending the whole day in the garden bending and digging after a winter of inactivity. This is not untypical of people in their middle age who have lost some physical strength and flexibility because of their lifestyle. They think that they can still do the things that they used to do 20 or 30 years earlier.

They may have a muscle tear or caused a problem and it is evident why it has happened. This problem is of no major concern. Yes the lack of mobility and pain is probably very unpleasant but the problem will be with them for a short period of time only.

At a later point they may have a further problem and it's usually, again, associated with something that they've done out of character from their normal lifestyle. They may think they have had a relapse of a back problem. It's not, it's just an additional episode of doing something for which they are either not strong enough, or over exerted themselves, or something they are not prepared for.

Chapter 2 – How to deal with relapses

Anybody who has had a major back problem and managed to cure themselves or had surgery will probably have some relapses. The initial reaction is one of utter devastation and possible terror thinking that it is another major attack.

Once you have reached the stage where your back is in good condition, following a major relapse, it is more likely to be a simple problem, which anyone could have had. The worry and stress is the biggest hurdle and one where you make things worse until you start to relax a little. If you have kept yourself in fairly good shape, are doing the daily exercises I've suggested and kept yourself flexible, your speed of recovery will be fast.

A standard statement my neurosurgeon always used to say was, if you have a really bad relapse "I'll allow you a maximum of a day in bed to feel sorry for yourself. After that, get up and start doing something."

It may hurt but just do it! There's no reason why you shouldn't get back on your feet very quickly. I occasionally have a minor relapse, I maybe twisted, I may be in a lot of pain. In reality, what's happened is I've not looked after myself well enough, I'm only human by the way, or I've moved something heavy I shouldn't have moved in a way that I knew I shouldn't have moved it. Hindsight is wonderful!

Get into the habit of looking after yourself sensibly, keep up with the exercises, and start doing the right things.

Major relapses

Many years ago I had a major back relapse that was absolutely horrifying. I had made such good progress and then all of a sudden my world was upside down again. I did get despondent for a while and thought things would never get better. Out of the darkness I started to think about what I could and should do. Quite simply, I went back to basics and considered what I had done the time before to get mobile again.

It is self-defeating to think it's useless because you will have the same problem again. Acknowledge what you've done, think about what you've not done that you should have done and tell yourself off. Then move forward.

I had people tell me it was pointless to carry on and try and get better as the same will happen again! These people had no place in my life and should have no place in yours – ask them to change their tune or leave you alone!

Remember, you are only human so ask some tough questions:

- Have you let yourself get out of condition?
- Have you stopped doing your exercises?
- Have you got a little lazy?
- Have you put on a little weight because you are less active?

Consider how you moved that cupboard or lifted those heavy items. Was it the wrong way because you were in a hurry? Perhaps you should have asked a neighbour to give you a hand but were too proud and thought you would do it yourself. The probability is your neighbour would have popped round and asked you, because they're not too proud....or they may not have asked and you have seen them hobbling around with a problem! Treat yourself as normal.

Importantly though, do try and think what caused the problem. It may not have been something you did yesterday. It may have been some of the things that you have not done over the previous few weeks. The cupboard you moved yesterday may not have been the major cause, it was just the final thing that has been compounded by many smaller things.

It may be a long car drive without getting out. It may be a long train journey or flight without doing some stretching. So, what haven't you been doing? What I have found from bitter personal experience is I've normally let myself slip and not considered some small things that have caused the problem.

Just to conclude this chapter I recommend that you quickly go back through this book and ask some questions:

- What am I not doing that I ought to?
- Have I forgotten my exercise regime?
- Have I put on weight?
- Am I eating the right things?
- Am I having the right amount of sleep?
- Am I travelling the best way – by car, train?
- Have I changed my car recently?
- When travelling do I stop for a short walk or get up every 90 minutes for a stretch?
- Have I been sitting with bad posture?
- Have I been sitting in the wrong type of seats?
- Have we had any new furniture that I am not sitting on properly?
- Have I started any new sport and it is only the initial aches?
- How much time am I spending watching television?
- How long do I sit without taking a break?
- Am I flexing enough?
- Am I actually de-stressing myself?
- Am I walking more and therefore the extra exercise is making me ache as part of getting better and fitter?
- Am I walking less?
- Have I just increased the amount of exercise I do by a significant margin?

Go right back to basics and work through – I am sure you will find things that you have started to do, or have slipped off your radar. Now is a good time to get back on track.

ACTION

- Commit to remaining positive if you have a relapse.

- Review what you do and have done that may have caused your relapse.

- Take remedial action if you can identify what you have done.

- Now continue with actions to restore mobility and reduce pain.

Chapter 3

Pain and the wider implications often overlooked

Medication

The first point of call for most people when they are suffering with back pain is to start taking painkillers. Initially this will be items that can be purchased over the counter at any pharmacy. The next stage is prescribed drugs, which are obtainable from your medical practitioner. Inevitably prescribed drugs will be stronger and will give relief from the extreme pain that back sufferers incur when they are having major problems.

The objective of everything that we shall be going through in this book is to minimise the level of pain that you experience so that the level of medication you need reduces. The ultimate goal will be to use no medication whatsoever on a routine basis. Crucially, there should be no dependency – it is sad to see people who have been taking medication for years and now treat it as a part of their lives. It does not have to be so!

A concern that everyone should have is forming a long-term dependency on back pain relieving medication. The key exception is where there is a chronic long-term problem with no way through to any form of self-healing. You need to challenge this if this is your problem. I don't want to raise false hopes but I remember to this day when I was told I would never walk again and probably be in a wheel chair at 50. I have taken delight in proving everyone wrong!

This level of dependency should be for far fewer people than many realise. So many people take the easy option of long-term medication as a way out, rather than develop ways to a better quality of life.

This last statement may seem cruel but it is a fact that far too many people 'make do' rather than get to the nub of the issue and get things sorted. So:

- Are you on medication?
- Do you need to be on medication?
- Really, do you need to be on medication?

Yes, a tough question but asking tough questions of ourselves and digging deep for the answer will make our longer term prospects so much better. Throughout this book there are significant things you can do to change your life ~ ultimately it is your choice.

I have seen people who have been prescribed morphine and got used to taking it – in spite of the pain I was in I did not, nor was I prescribed drugs for more than a brief period of time. I saw the ease of becoming dependent....... that was no life for me, I am sure it is no life for you either!

I had a very major problem and my medical practitioner did prescribe some drugs early on. I was committed to being pain free and medication free so quickly stopped taking them and 'listened' to what my body told me. Some people are less fortunate and their medical practitioner keeps prescribing strong drugs. My advice is to take ownership as many of the decisions can be yours. I worked hard to be pain free and medication free.

'Cold turkey'

Please take note that if you have been on prescribed drugs for a period of time you will need to 'wean' yourself off them. If you have been on morphine for any period of time you cannot just stop else you will get what is casually called 'cold turkey'. This is where you will have withdrawal symptoms if you suddenly stop, so do be careful. You need to speak to your medical practitioner and explain what you are doing so they can help you reduce and then eliminate your dependency.

Hope to Cope

A major concern I have is that many people live a life of coping rather than take the opportunity to create a life where back pain and problems are resolved. This becomes a self-fulfilling wish because all they will do is cope with their situation rather than take a positive approach to moving forward. Many people will just hope that things will get better – things may, but it is far better to take a proactive approach to regaining better health and take control of your situation. So please take matters into your own hands using this book to take you away from the 'hope to cope' philosophy and to a proactive approach taking responsibility for your own welfare and health.

Effect

As anyone with serious back pain will know, the debilitating effects of this pain are appalling. This covers a number of factors:

- The first is obviously the pain itself, which causes people to flinch and cry out, just with the terrible pain which this ailment causes.
- In some extreme cases it stops people completing even the most basic tasks as the pain level is so intense.
- The loss of mobility caused through the pain and spasm can and does totally change lives – in some cases instantly.

Anything beyond the merest level of survival is just not possible. For those people who live with, and for those that care for people with significant back pain, it is all too obvious, and needs no further explanation.

Chapter 3 – Pain and the wider implications often overlooked

Some of the less obvious initial effects of back pain are slow to manifest themselves but are significant. These include:

- Looking drained.
- Having low energy levels.
- In some cases losing weight.
- Starting to give up.
- Not taking care of ourselves.
- Not dressing properly.
- Not engaging in anything.
- Watching more TV or in some cases no longer watching TV but doing nothing instead.
- Not speaking as much.
- Moaning.
- Being edgy.

The daily challenge of just combating pain, which may not be suppressed by medication, means that there is a slow but inevitable toll on the person's body, and enthusiasm for life.

On a broader front the effects impact upon every aspect of a person's life. This will include:

- Family
- Friends
- Relationships
- Work
- Hobbies
- Sport
- And any other activity that the person formerly undertook.

The impact that this has physically is one side of the coin, the other side is the impact that this has mentally. Therefore when dealing with back pain it is vital not to start on a downward spiral, which could result in depression. In addition, the wish to do anything starts to diminish and therefore this too can become a downward spiral and life loses it spark and fun.

For those who are close to people with back pain this is where care and consideration are required to support the person through a difficult time. Do bear in mind that relationships may end up becoming quite strained. At worse the person who is supporting appears to become nagging and the person in pain is seen to be lazy and uninterested in getting better. For the person directly involved it is important that some activities are undertaken to stimulate some self-confidence and self-worth. Maintaining the will to find a way out of the situation that you are in and at least seeing some value in even small steps and activities are vital. There is always something you can do.

Referred Pain

The body is a strange thing as pain in one area can easily be referred to another part of the body. One may find that an intense painful muscular spasm in the upper left side of the back may in fact have been caused by a problem in the lower right hand side or somewhere else altogether. An important part of starting to self treat one's back is to acknowledge that what may appear to be the source of pain could in fact be elsewhere – **this is a key point**.

As an example I once met someone who was clearly in pain and they were rubbing their upper right shoulder – the source of the problem was tension just below the left shoulder blade. This is not an unusual case where the cause of the pain was elsewhere so do 'explore' where the source of the pain may be coming from.

It is therefore important to start to make notes of where pain starts from, plus the impact on other parts of the body. This can be tied into the measurement of your pain and the change in lifestyle, which is referred to in chapter 13. It is a very useful process to keep this recorded at the same time as your daily measurements also referred to in chapter 13. So keep a daily log of key aspects of your current condition. I would suggest that these are just the odd sentence or a few bullet point notes and not a full essay per day. You are aiming to build up a log of your problem – in essence a reference file. This can be in a diary, a separate note book, or a ring binder.

I kept a log of my problems and some days I wrote very little, whilst on other days I wrote much more. You will determine what works for you but do record this information – it is valuable. On the days when you are feeling particularly low, it is probably more important than ever so set yourself the challenge of keeping this daily log.

Effects on other parts of the body

One of the surprising aspects of back pain is the impact that it can have on other parts of your body.

- A painful and twisted back will have significant effect on the ability to breathe properly. Breathing will become shallow. The resulting effect is that the body is not getting as much oxygen as it normally would when normal or deeper breaths are being taken. This in itself is a problem because it will create lethargy and also the all important flow of well-oxygenated blood to parts of the body that need repairing will be affected.
- Other symptoms from a twisted painful back could mean that one's stomach feels uncomfortable and eating is less easy.
- It could mean that the gut is twisted and therefore normal bodily functions are less comfortable.
- A fairly typical problem with people with back problems is if they can walk they will start to walk in a very awkward way. Instead of feet pointing forward at 12 o'clock or five to twelve it is not uncommon for the feet to point out at ten to two or extreme cases quarter to three. This will cause a problem with leg muscles. They will be used in a way which is uncomfortable and causes additional tension.

- If one's back is not vertical, and perhaps skewed to the left or right hand side, in order to see straight in front compensation will be needed in one's neck. As you can well imagine this will start to create stresses and strains in the neck, resulting in additional aches.
- In bad cases of back problems the lower spine bulges in the wrong direction causing the person to walk with a stoop so that the shoulders are slumped forward and this will cause other aches because of poor posture. Often the shoulders are also misaligned with one being much lower than the other.

I mention this to highlight some of the significant impacts a bad back can have elsewhere in one's body. This inevitably starts to cause an increase in aches and pains in other seemingly unrelated parts of one's body. No wonder we can feel dreadful! It is all part of the impact back pain can inflict.

So the impact of having a back problem could cause other problems to start as your body is making compensations. In the short term this is not a major issue, albeit do note the changes you are making. In the longer term this could start to create serious changes in your body, leading to other problems.

Don't get frightened by this but do note that awareness is a key part of the process of making steps to regain healthy ways.

SUMMARY

- So where is your pain?
- What other parts of your body are being affected?
- What impact is this having?
- Am I starting to keep a daily log and make simple notes about where it hurts?
- Am I thinking about areas of my body other than my back too?
- How am I treating others?

- How cheerful am I or am I just downright miserable?
- Have I eaten well today?
- What is my breathing like?

ACTION

- Be truthful about any medication you take – prescribed and other. List them all down with the aim to reduce and then exclude as many as you can.

- Start a log to register the pain levels.

- Think about where your pain is – be as detailed as you can and log this information down so you can review progress over time.

- Be clear about the impact pain is having on you and your world, e.g. your work, your home life.

Chapter 4

Food and Drink: The impact on recovery speed

Introduction to section

There is not one area that will solve a back problem. It is a build up of many things that all make a difference. A difference that when combined with other things help make the difference between being healthy and fit or continuing to be debilitated.

The area of food and drink is a critical piece of the jigsaw that will aid rehabilitation.

You may say, "I eat well already." If that is the case this section will only be a confirmation of what you do. If you say I love my food and drink and it is the only thing that makes the pain bearable, the treats during the day, the glass of something that helps with the pain.......I would suggest you take serious note of this section – it may just change your life.

What you eat

The essence behind diet is to ensure that you are getting the right amount and right type of food without increasing your weight, unless you are very thin. It is important that your back is not carrying excessive weight, which is a burden and strains the very part of your body that you are trying to repair.

If you are honest with yourself you will know what weight you should be. And I mean really honest – the only person you are fooling if you are not, is yourself. If you think you are big boned, your family is always heavy and any other such excuses stop yourself now. Acknowledge that they are excuses – now decide to do something about your weight and health.

I do stress that the temptation to sit and eat comforting foods is very real when you are in pain. It is a distraction and it gives you a short term feel good factor. The problem is that the most convenient and comforting food may be full of fat and sugar – neither of which are helpful to your recovery. In fact they are counterproductive. They will increase your weight. They will also start to impede the flow of blood, which is critical in the healing process associated with back problems. And probably mess up your digestion, as you are getting no proper exercise. A tough comment, but true.

Meal time

It may sound obvious but it is wise to eat at regular intervals. Do have breakfast at a "normal" time and the same with lunch and dinner. Committing to having a sensible time plan is valuable.

Make the effort to get up even though it may be very painful and have breakfast as a proper first meal of the day. This does not mean a large fry up. If you are not doing much exercise you will not need as much fuel to keep you going so do be sensible. You should be eating relatively little fat and sugar. That is deliberate. This is part of a balanced and positive approach to getting you back on your feet, after being so debilitated. Another critical part of about getting up, and having breakfast at an early enough time, is it will create a discipline to get your body moving. Every temptation is to lie in bed for just a little bit longer. **The only reason to slob around in your dressing gown and pyjamas all day is laziness.** The activity of actually getting up and getting going is a crucial part of starting to create a life that is more active than the one you are currently experiencing.

This is also a major part of ensuring at the start of the day you are fuelling yourself with high quality food which will start to increase the probability of you getting back on your feet, and living a more mobile life than you currently have.

I hear of people who stay in bed till late morning, someone bringing their breakfast in bed, and then they rest for a little longer before they get up. This is a serious error and will only make things worse. Ideally, having breakfast in bed should be avoided – it is far better to eat breakfast at a table once you have showered (shaved if a man) and dressed.

Snacks

In between meals there will be a tendency to want to snack. This is sometimes because there is nothing else to do if you are sitting in pain and unable to move easily. It is a pleasant distraction just to nibble something to while away the time and give you something to do. To take your mind off things. There is a real danger that friends and family will bring you nice little treats to help you get better. They mean well but in many cases what they bring will be counterproductive to restoring your health. Examples such as:

- Nuts
- Biscuits
- Cake
- Crisps
- Chocolates
- Cream cakes
- Danish pastries
- Ice cream

They all seem very nice and very innocent. BUT do bear in mind that nuts, crisps, cake and chocolate are very high in fat and are some of the **most** calorific foods you can eat.

Often visitors may say that they have called in with their pastry and use the teasing words "go on it won't hurt you to share".

They are active, you are not, so resist temptation – explain the truth and ask them to help by not tempting you.

During a normal day and evening it is easy to consume more than twice your ideal calorie intake just by nibbling away on comfort food and tit bits. Think, most nuts are over 60% fat, some are close to 80% fat and over 700 calories per 100g!

Get used to reading food labels so you can assess the calorific value.

Another thing to be mindful of if you are whiling away your time watching TV or a film is the association with familiar habits. There can be a conditioned link – Film = Treats to nibble. Be very careful of habits. Still to this day if I go to see a film I want popcorn, and the sticky variety because that is what we did as children with our parents.

I am not being a killjoy and saying don't have snacks between meals. What I am saying is be **very** selective about what you do eat. As guidance I have given a few examples below of good and bad things to eat.

Good:
Raw vegetables such as carrot, celery, radish
Fruit in moderation
Low fat yogurt
Popcorn with no salt or sugar coating
Small amounts of dried fruit

Bad:
Most nuts
Chocolate
Cakes and biscuits
Crisps
Pies
Pizza
Take away meals

Yogurts unless low fat
Ice cream
White grapes

If you are someone who is easily tempted into eating items on the bad list, I suggest you ask people not to give you the temptation in the first place and don't bring anything – a form of tough love. People do like to bring something on occasion when visiting so if they ask, request a magazine or just say that you are delighted they want to come and their company is all you want.

There is a preconditioned feeling that if we are seeing someone who is not well that we ought to take something for them. I strongly recommend that you lay out the ground rules right from the start. If you are reading this book and have been immobile for a while, now is a great time to set out new rules. You have the opportunity of a new start so take it.

Lunch

By the time lunchtime has arrived it becomes a welcome distraction into the day. This is particularly so for people who are very immobile. For those who are more active it is vital that more food is eaten to refuel the body. I have found from personal experience if you try and skip lunch you end up eating snacks that are both inappropriate and also have far more calories than a decent lunch. The best advice is always to have fresh light food and avoid all of the heavy comfort food. If it is cold, a light but hot soup is always a good choice avoiding added cream and butter.

Dinner

This is the last meal of the day and an opportunity to eat something that is really enjoyable and appropriate in creating another small step on your road to more mobility. I do stress that this is not an opportunity to catch up on all of the missed opportunities from the day and have a large "feast". The objective is to have something that is very satisfying and allows you to go to bed not feeling bloated or full. I would recommend that you eat your last meal at least 2 hours before going to bed and not to 'graze' on little titbits after dinner either.

I have found that whilst it may be easier to eat somewhere you consider to be "comfortable and cosy" it is much better to eat at a table. Avoid eating off a tray on your knee at all costs. This is for a number of reasons:

- Whilst the chair at the table may appear to be less comfortable it will generally create a better posture.
- Having your meal at a table is better because it is flat, stable and less likely to require you to hunch or curve your back in a way that you would if you were sitting in that comfortable chair looking at the television.
- It helps your digestive system. Your stomach will be less twisted and bunched up. If you are hunched up on the sofa you are really making it tough for your digestion.
- It enables you to have a glass of water within reach so you can keep well hydrated. Do drink the water too.
- It encourages you to use proper eating techniques that allow you to feel "human and normal" again.
- It gives you support with a firm table should you have a spasm of pain.
- It provides a solid and firm surface from which to rise, so that you can start to walk.
- It makes you move from where you were and in itself is an active form of exercise.
- This regular journey, whilst painful at times, will encourage movement which is vital for increasing the health and strength of your back.
- It enables proper discussion with anyone at home in a way that is conducive to creating a conversation less about you and more about your family, friends and life in general. Make the focus anything but you.

- It takes your mind elsewhere which will divert you from thinking about the pain and suffering that you are going through.
- It shows other people that you are trying to get better.

As a summary for the type of food I would always stress:

- Buy and eat the best and freshest that is available.
- Eat seasonal fruit and vegetables – they tend to be fresher and travelled less to get to your table.
- Eat lean meat in preference to fatty – choose smaller better cuts.
- Remove excess fat from all foods.
- Minimise the amount of saturated fat you eat.
- Keep salt levels down to the recommended level.
- Aim to avoid processed foods.
- Use natural products rather than synthetic.
- Read food labels – you may be shocked by what you have been eating!

Drink

You need to keep your body well hydrated to give it the best chance to heal. If you are wrapped up warm, or it is a hot day you will be losing fluid through perspiration and the very act of breathing – our breath is very humid. Also if you are in pain it is not unusual to have 'cold sweats'. You are losing fluid.

It may be painful to get up to go to the toilet, so you are less inclined to drink. Do not use this as an excuse not to drink! There are other problems that you can store up if you drink too little. To put an indicator down regarding volume is difficult due to our size, the heat, our pain levels and other factors – the easy way to confirm that you are drinking enough is to make sure your urine is almost colourless. If it is yellow you are not drinking enough.

Non-Alcoholic

Avoid caffeine-based drinks. Caffeine is in coffee, tea, cola drinks and surprisingly in chocolate drinks.

Why? Caffeine reduces the size of capillaries, which are the very small blood vessels, which enable the blood supply to reach every part of the body. This is important as capillaries primarily feed the blood flow to the area around the spine. If the blood supply is struggling to get to these difficult to reach part of the body there is less opportunity for it to do its healing work.

This means that if you are used to drinking large amounts of tea and coffee, you may find it quite a challenge. There are caffeine free alternatives:

- Redbush tea – very similar to 'normal' tea
- Herbal teas

Tip – don't force yourself to drink herbal teas you don't like by filling them full of sugar, find ones you do like and aim to be sugar free.

Tip – for tea use soya or skimmed milk rather than full fat milk. Avoid stir-in whitening powders as they are usually highly processed and high in fat.

Generally aim to avoid decaffeinated tea or coffee – the caffeine is often removed by a chemical process.

I have heard of people having withdrawal symptoms when they stop drinking coffee. I suggest you take note of how you feel, but do aim to remove caffeine drinks from your lifestyle as quickly as possible. I have also heard of people who feel so much better when they stop drinking tea and coffee that they never go back to it. Interesting!

My suggestion if you are struggling to stop drinking tea or coffee, is to have a cup of your favourite tea or coffee once a day as a treat and drink the alternatives the rest of the day. When I was making the transition I would choose to have coffee made from freshly ground beans for my mid morning treat.

Soft Drinks

Generally these contain a large amount of sugar. Part of a healthy diet is minimising the amount of refined food that you are consuming. Drinks such as squashes, fizzy drinks, colas and "juice drinks" all contain refined sugar or a synthetic low calorie sweetening additive (that does not sound very pleasant does it?) so treat these with considerable caution. They have limited use in restoring your health.

Do drink lots of water, still is better because if you drink carbonated water your body has to deal with the carbon dioxide that you are drinking in the bubbles. At this time your body has enough to be getting on with without this additional demand.

Fruit Juices

Fruit juices are fine and a valuable part of a good diet. They contain natural sugars so a responsible approach to the amount that you drink during the course of each day is important. Do consider the acid content though as you don't want to upset your stomach. Also just be a little careful, as an excessive amount of fruit juice without active dental hygiene and care could mean that there will be a detrimental impact on your teeth.

Initially it may taste a little odd but a good way of drinking wisely is to dilute fruit juices with water.

Alcoholic Drinks

There is a temptation when you are in a lot of pain to try and reduce the pain by drinking alcoholic beverages. This is not good news, for a number of reasons:

- You are consuming a large amount of calories which is not good for general health.
- You are trying to hide pain in a way which does not allow you to deal with it properly.
- You will become less lucid and the conversation with the people around you will be very superficial – they may also get tired of you being in a stupor and wallowing in an alcoholic haze. Perversely, alcohol can cause wakefulness even if initially it leads to dozing.
- You will smell of alcohol – which is never very pleasant for non drinkers. Especially children.
- The time you start to drink will slowly get earlier in the day.
- This is in addition to the obvious health risks of over drinking that are well documented in many other places. E.g. dehydration and lowering of blood sugar levels.

It could be your choice of avoiding alcoholic drinks completely. The risky times are meal times such as lunch and dinner, and a night cap at the end of the day. I believe a small alcoholic drink taken as a relaxant has its part to play but only in certain circumstances.

My recommendation is to avoid alcohol altogether for the time being – it is so easy for it to become a regular part of your daily ritual that you try and justify. It is far wiser to have the occasional drink (be sensible!) and fully enjoy it. This means it does not become an addictive part of your own method of pain control. It is also something that you can look forward to once you are fit and well again.

If you do choose to have a drink of wine my recommendation is to avoid white wine and stick with red. The reason behind this is that it has been found that white wine has a tendency to exacerbate arthritis and the symptoms associated with arthritis such as achy joints and stiffness. Red wine does not have the same drawbacks as white wine. It is generally drunk more moderately than white too. The simple reason is that chilled white wine (how most of us drink white wine) tends to slip down all too easily on a hot summer day. Or when we open the first bottle – often because we are thirsty rather than intending to drink large amounts. A simple tip is to always drink water before you drink wine and also have a glass of water on the table at the same time.

Many people enjoy spirits, a beer or a lager, which are also fine in moderation but be warned of the high calorific value these drinks have. This may seem as if I am being highly critical of alcoholic drinks – I am not but it is so easy when suffering with back pain to use it as a way of easing the pain or as a distraction. Therefore the risk of sitting or lying around, doing very little but drinking and eating large amounts, increases body weight. This in turn becomes a real problem as it places more strain on an already painful back.

Another major problem of alcohol is it sends you to sleep so you end up living a very inactive life that only adds to the problems you already have. Remember when you have been sober and speaking to someone who has been drinking, it is clear that they are 'not always with it'. You may become quite boring and intolerable even with small amounts of alcohol.

It can be so tempting to have a sleep after a heavy meal or an alcoholic drink too (the combination makes it all the more tempting). A further problem is if you fall asleep in a chair you will almost certainly place a strain on some part of your spine – not good news.

As a final point, be warned about the implications of drinking alcohol with any form of medication you have been prescribed, or are taking. Usually they don't mix!

Smoking

Quite simple, be a non-smoker. If you smoke you will reduce the amount of oxygen into your body, oxygen that is needed in healing. You will reduce the size of your capillaries (blood vessels) and it will take longer to heal.

My advice – invest the money you save into good quality food.

Supplements

This is an area where some people believe supplements have an active and valuable part to play in our diet. Some believe they are just a fad and are unnecessary. My view is that anything that helps restore a healthy body is valuable and worthy of consideration.

Mass and intense farming has reduced the amount of vitamins and minerals contained in our foods. It is therefore worth considering adding some supplements to your diet. My recommendation is quite simple:

- 1 good quality multivitamin and mineral formula per day
- 250mg of vitamin C twice per day. One in the morning with breakfast and one with dinner in the early evening.

NOTE: As always though, before embarking on any form of self-medication, do discuss this with your medical practitioner. In this case you may also wish to consider seeing a nutritionist who will be able to advise on what suits you best. Most supplements are easily obtained on the High Street.

Use the activity of meal times as a part of your self-treatment. Get involved with preparing for your eating and drinking. You may really struggle to do any activity whatsoever and the thought of getting out of bed, or getting out of that comfortable chair seems an effort because it creates additional pain. This is something that I consider to be a significant part of taking responsibility for your journey back to full health. If you live by yourself you have to do it. If you have other people about make the effort and don't be lazy because someone else is at hand.

Getting up at a sensible time to prepare breakfast is a first step on that journey. Going to bed at a sensible time is important too.

This next statement may sound tough – If you are supported by your family and friends and they insist upon looking after you and getting all your meals I will guarantee that your speed of recovery will be massively lengthened.

Take an active part even if it is only a small initial step. At every meal time, for every drink and for every snack you need to earn the reward. Start and then continue on the road to your recovery.

The effort of having to get into the kitchen and do something starts to create mobility and is all part of the process of regaining your life. Yes, it will be tough. You may even have to crawl into the kitchen when you are suffering with massive pain but do it!

- The bending to get something out of the fridge is valuable exercise.
- The reaching to get something out of a cupboard is valuable exercise.
- The standing by the sink to prepare something is valuable exercise.

Don't convince yourself that you are in so much pain and cannot do it. You can if you are determined enough. If people around you insist on doing everything for you, be firm with them and insist they don't. This is tough but believe me, they are steps worth taking. **If the people around you cannot bear to see you struggle, ask them to leave the room or go for a short walk so they don't see you in pain.**

It may be that to get to the kitchen you need a stool or something placed part way so that you can have a rest on the journey.

Perhaps something to rest on while you are part way through what seems like a simple task. It is better to do the task in stages even though it causes you significant pain and discomfort. Refer to the section on furniture for additional thoughts on this area too.

Teeth – it has been mentioned briefly above but do take care of your dental hygiene and as a minimum keep your teeth brushed morning and night. The last thing you want is toothache to add to your problems!

One final point regarding food and drink – take total responsibility for everything that you eat and drink. Play an active part in the choices of menus, the types of food and drink that you consume. Especially if you are not the key person that prepares these in your household. It is your responsibility, your pain and your opportunity to reclaim a more fulfilling life so do not delegate, or abdicate this to anyone else.

ACTION

- Review what you eat and drink

- What changes are you now going to implement into your diet?

- Where do you currently eat your meals? Now commit to eating main meals at a table.

- Say 'NO' to the wrong treats.

- Stop smoking.

- Let people around you know what changes are being made and why. Ask them to help and explain what they need to do to help you have a healthy diet.

Chapter 5

Taking a sensible approach to fitness

NOTE: *Always consult your medical practitioner before undertaking any exercises.* Act responsibly and if excessive pain or strain is experienced in attempting any of the actions explained in this book or if anyone is under medical supervision, it is recommended to follow the advice of their doctor, medical practitioner or physiotherapist.

This section will not cover sporting activities. It will focus on the initial areas and subsequent regime to lay the foundations for a basic level of back fitness. It will include an initial series of simple exercises that should be incorporated into a daily routine to start to treat a back problem. Then secondly, once the back problem has started to be controlled and movement increases, a maintenance regime will be proposed.

Exercise regime – getting you started

In the very early stages of a major back problem, which usually creates significant spasms in the back, it is tough to do anything. The initial reaction is to do nothing. This is generally the wrong thing to do. Although initially, just to combat the shock and possible terror of the pain and loss of mobility, simply resting for a period of time may be the right thing for you. Crucially, do not let this period of time become too long – and this means hours or the odd day. What I propose may seem totally counter intuitive but it is recommended that movement, even if small, is started after the first few hours of immobility.....you did read that right, hours!

I had a major problem many years before the episode that made me write this book. Bed rest was prescribed at the time so I spent two weeks in bed. It was awful and quickly my muscles lost their strength. It took a long time to get back to any level of fitness. Also it was difficult to regain my balance as I had been used to no movement and I felt 'light headed' when I stood up. The current thoughts are to get active. My specialist said at most 12 hours in bed before I should get mobile, preferably less!

It will require a lot of determination to do even simple things but the effort of doing anything that you can, at this stage, will be well rewarded.

If you are in bed or in a chair the first thing to do is lie on the floor. (Do not lie on a hard cold floor though; make sure that it has a carpet or a rug on it.) I know this in itself will be a major and potentially painful event but this is the starting point for a series of simple exercises to start to help you on your road to recovery. **Before you do this though – ensure that you can get back up again from the floor.** So ensure that a solid piece of furniture is reasonably close by or you have access to one or two sticks that you can use to help yourself off the floor after these exercises have been undertaken. Also, for the first few times when doing the exercises until you gain some confidence it may be worth having someone who can help you within earshot.

Typically, I would always carry a phone with me if I knew I was going to get into a situation where I may experience some new challenge. Do make sure it is well charged and you have a signal.

WARNING these exercises are not intended to be forced in any way so only do what is possible but be assured that anything at this stage will be better than nothing. It is not a contest and don't treat it as one.

If any of these exercises exaggerate the back pain, then they should not be performed.

Exercise 1

Floor lying.

Quite simply lie on your back and aim to stretch your legs out in front of you on the floor – so you are simply just lying on the floor. Start to try and relax letting your body go as limp as possible and acknowledging where the pain is coming from. Try and be specific and make a mental note, which you should write down later. Let your mind relax too and try and think of nothing.

Exercise 2

Straightening out.

If you are twisted so that your upper body is not aligned with your legs start to try and straighten yourself so that your body is straight. Do **not** force what clearly is not meant to be though! It is much better to do this in stages with a small adjustment each time, this is far better than trying to do too much too soon and setting yourself further back.

Exercise 3

Knees raised floor twists.

Slowly and carefully bend one leg and slide your foot so your heel is aligned with the knee of the leg that is flat on the floor. Now move the other leg into the same position. You should now be lying on the floor your knees together with your feet flat on the floor. The shape that this makes with your legs will be similar to a triangle. If you need help to raise your legs do use your hands. If you need to support your legs to help with the pain then do so.

Now slowly lower your two legs together to the left. If they manage to reach the floor that is fine, if they don't that is also fine – don't force them. During this part of the exercise you are aiming to keep your shoulders as flat as possible on the floor. If you find this very difficult, support your legs as they start to lower with your hand. So if you are leaning your legs to the left support with your left hand, and vice versa for the right.

Now raise your knees from whatever position they reached back to the vertical central position i.e. where you started. Now lower your knees in the opposite direction following the same rules as just mentioned. This is one stretch, made up of two parts.

The object of this exercise is to introduce a gentle twist between your lower and upper body that will place a stretch into the opposite part of your back. Hold each stretch for a few seconds but do not force the stretch or endure too much pain during this exercise. It is suggested that you start with five stretches. If you can only manage one, that is better than none, and stop after just one. If you find this exercise reasonably easy I suggest you do a maximum of ten stretches to each side. The objective for everyone is to work to a maximum of ten stretches each side.

Exercise 4

Sit ups (crunches).

Yes, I am being serious! Still in the position of lying on the floor with your knees bent, aim to raise your shoulders and head off the floor by about 15 centimetres (6 inches). Initially keep your hands in front of you on the floor and let them slide forward as you complete each sit up. Only aim to do a few to start with, say 5. If you can only manage one, try for two. Eventually aim to do 25. To make this exercise more powerful, eventually aim to place your hands behind your head to do this exercise. As with all exercises do not strain and start slowly. If it means you can only raise your shoulders and head off the floor by 5 centimetres initially that is fine. As I said at the beginning of this section, this is not a contest.

Exercise 5

Back bridge.

Keep your feet and legs still in the pyramid position lying on the floor. The objective of this exercise is to raise your bottom off the floor so that your thighs and back form one straight line down to your shoulders. Do not strain yourself doing this exercise. If you are suffering badly with back pain this exercise will prove tough. Do not let this deter you. The best way to do this for the first time is to place your elbows at your side, ease your hands under your bottom and use your hands to raise your bottom into the air. Also use your hands to lower your bottom to the ground. Hold each raise initially for only one or two seconds, the objective being to work up to ten seconds. The number of repeats for this exercise is recommended at a maximum of ten but if you find this tough one initially is fine. If you are very weak or well overweight don't over exert yourself.

Next.

Now lower your legs to the floor and take a moment or two to settle your body again.

When you are ready, roll over from your back onto your front. You may find that using your hands or even a piece of furniture helps this too. If the pain is high the only way to achieve this is by 'trial and error'. Don't get disheartened as there will be a way and the effort is all part of the journey. If you are 'too round' to lie comfortably flat on your front there is a message here and something to also work on.

Exercise 6

Alternate rear leg lifts.

Lying on your front, rest your arms bent at shoulder height and place your hands under your chin. Once comfortable, or as comfortable as you think you can get, slowly lift one leg up in the air about 15 centimetres (6 inches) and then gently lower. Now do the same with the opposite leg. Aim to complete 15 repetitions, in turn, with each leg. At first you may only manage a few and you may not manage to lift to the recommended height. A small start is better than no start and you must not force yourself too hard. Likewise, don't give up too soon.

Exercise 7

Trunk curls.

Still lying on your front, your objective is to raise your torso from the floor with your hands behind your back. Aim to raise your shoulders off the floor by 22 centimetres (9 inches). This IS a strong exercise and initially may be impossible so don't try too hard if it is. A simple way to get things moving though is to place your hands flat with palms down under each shoulder and gently help by pressing with your arms, much in the same way that you would with a press-up. Only your torso should rise from the floor, as you are aiming to bend from the waist upwards. If your hips start to rise from the floor you are doing the exercise wrong, or over exerting, and may have to limit the height your shoulders rise to only a small height, say 5 – 10 centimetres (2 or 3 inches). Don't feel defeated, it will improve in good time. Your goal is 25.

Exercise 8

Press-ups.

This is a strong exercise for back sufferers but one that is important in the medium term. Always start doing these in a modest way and never strain. There is a difference between pain and over exerting oneself. The best way to start is to lie on one's front, and with hands at shoulder height, palms down gently press upwards so your arms become straight. Initially only do press up from your knees. In the fullness of time you can do these from your feet so your whole body is straight. It is always best to start from the knee position and raise yourself as high as you can. When starting also do not always aim to straighten your arms. The ultimate aim is 10 repetitions but start with only as many as you can manage.

Exercise 9

Child pose.

Once you have finished these exercises, a wonderful final position is to end up in the yoga posture called 'The Child'. This is where you start in the kneeling position, then lower you bottom so you are sitting on your legs and then lower your torso over your thighs so you head is resting on the floor. This is a big stretch position and will pull on your spine. As always don't overdo it and if you can get into the position relax into it for a few minutes. Don't stay too long as you may stiffen up and find it difficult to unravel.

Frequency – it is recommended that these exercises are undertaken first thing in the morning and again in the evening. Also during the initial recovery stage it is a good idea to do them halfway through the day as well.

NOTE:

It is better to do a few and regularly rather than too many at only one time. Don't overdo it. You may be quite competitive and feel that you must do the maximum possible. If you force yourself beyond a reasonable level you will set yourself back so be sensible and build up slowly and surely.

Maintenance

Even when one's back is no longer causing a problem it is wise to undertake these exercises on a regular basis. Ideally these should be completed in the morning and the evening seven days a week. As a compromise, once per day for six days will be fine once you are fit again. I would suggest that these exercises become part of your daily routine and a sure way to keep your back stronger. Should you have any future problems you will recover much quicker than if you have let them lapse. As a guide they should take 5 – 10 minutes only once you are well again.

Other opportunities

All opportunities should be taken to start to regain fitness as soon as possible following a major back episode. Seemingly simple things such as climbing the stairs should be used to start to create fitness and an increase in mobility in back health. It is easy to avoid doing things because you know it will hurt. Yes, it is easy to ask someone to fetch something from upstairs that you have forgotten or you need. Use it as an opportunity as it will start to increase your mobility and remove the excuse that because it hurts you cannot do it. It is easy to change the channel of a television with a remote handset, do not use this as an excuse to sit and be lazy and not do anything. Take the opportunity when you have finished watching television to turn it off at the set. So get up and do it. If you want anything from anywhere else in the house aim to get up and get it. It may be easier for others around you to be supportive and get what you need but it is a false economy on your journey to an improved quality of life and helping cure your back problem.

An observation

If you have been inactive for any period of time or are generally unfit you may start to ache after exercise. There is a balance here between an ache because you have done some exercise and a pain because you have overdone things.

Consider what it would be like if you decided after 20 years of inactivity to head off down the gym for the first time. If you do much at all you're going to come back and ache. It's a fairly natural thing that would happen. If you go for a long walk at the weekend, having not been on one for two or three years you'll probably ache. If you decide on holiday you're going to run down the beach a few times you're probably going to ache. That is normal and that is what was happening to you.

When I started to exercise I ached terribly on top of the pain I was suffering, it seemed to make things worse. I initially thought this is horrible but reconsidered and then realised where the extra aches were coming from and knew I had to continue. I had reached a point where I was pushing myself into the pain before the gain. I understood the balance between doing too little and doing too much – sometimes by trial and painful error! Doing nothing was not an option and each activity gave me the opportunity to take the next step.

A thought

If you have been generally unfit this may be one of the reasons you now have a back problem. Take heart in the fact that these exercises will help you start on a journey back to better overall health too.

ACTION

- Start your exercise regime – slowly at first – is now a good time to start?

- Keep a daily schedule and record when you did your exercises.

- Record each exercise and the repetitions you do each time.

- Review the progress you are making.

- What other actions could you do that others currently are doing for you?

Chapter 6

Remaining active and even taking up a new sport

> *NOTE: Always consult your medical practitioner before undertaking any exercises.* Act responsibly and if excessive pain or strain is experienced in attempting any of the actions explained in this book or if anyone is under medical supervision, it is recommended to follow the advice of their doctor, medical practitioner or physiotherapist.

If you are used to playing a sport on a regular basis it will come as something of a shock when you are unable to carry on due to a major back problem. The objective we have is to ensure that you are back to health so that you can resume any sporting activity that you have previously undertaken.

If you are not a sporty person now could be a good opportunity to start to think about what you could undertake that will get you active and starting to use your body as nature intended. It may seem ridiculous at this stage especially if you have had a major back episode but I can assure you that where there is a will there should be a way.

If you are not a sporting person and wondering what you could start to do I have listed below a few options and the reasons behind why I think they are suitable. There is a variety and some of them may seem a little extreme. Also I have selected some which will fit a number of budgets. You don't need to compete, only participate.

Swimming

An easy activity as most towns have a public swimming pool. It is a good all round exercise and as the water supports your weight it is not as hard as some activities. It is always advisable to mention to the lifeguard that you have a back problem so they can respond quickly if you need to have help, and often they will help you get out if you are having a few problems. A tip – take a walking stick with you to the pool side as it will help you from slipping on the wet floor, other people will also see you have a problems and be more careful. Try and visit the pool at quiet times so that you are not competing with others for space.

If you can't swim, now could be a great time to learn. There are classes at most pools for most age groups and is nothing to be embarrassed about, in fact quite the reverse and you should be proud to start to learn.

General walking

The easiest activity you can take as it starts at your front door. Start slowly and build up. Change your route and incorporate a hill or two as you improve. Do look at the ground you are walking on as a small undulation in the past would not have been an issue. With a serious back problem even the smallest unevenness can be a surprise and a painful challenge. If possible never use a stick as it will either create dependence or 'skew' how you walk. I do advise taking a short stick to show others that you have a problem until you feel more secure.

If you need a stick I suggest you use two. I explain the reason below.

Chapter 6 – Remaining active and even taking up a new sport

Hill walking

This is the next stage on from general walking. It does not need to be mountain trekking with lots of specialist equipment. It is a case of choosing more challenging terrain from general walking. This may also mean that the type of footwear may need to be sturdier. With uneven terrain it may be wise to use walking poles. You may have seen people walking with a pole, or two poles that are quite long. These are the best sort, albeit walking sticks are also fine, if the ground is not too steep. I would always advocate using two poles – it may look a bit silly but forget that. The reason two are better than one is that they will provide support both sides, it is easier to steady yourself if you feel unstable and it avoids twisting that occurs when people use only one. The use of poles is a chapter in its own right but I am sure you get the gist!

Gym

There are gyms everywhere at very different prices. If you want the club feeling it will cost more than the down to earth ones. Remember this is not about body building just about developing a better level of posture and muscle tone to help in daily life – so avoid the ones targeting body building. There is usually a good personal fitness trainer available to help create a routine of appropriate exercises. If they do not understand back problems try another gym. If they are keen on increasing the weights and resistance be very sceptical. You are not trying to 'bulk up' you are seeking flexibility with sufficient strength – so use increased repetitions not weight.

The first gym I tried seemed very helpful but the level of weight was higher than I felt was right and the repetitions were lower so I changed to someone who had a better understanding. Forget the 'macho' image. I frequently had to adjust equipment from 80kg down to 20kg and whilst I may have lost face with some people that is their concern not mine. Someone I know insisted on using heavy weights to cure his back problem, thinking bulk and strength were the right things – he hobbles on two sticks, I don't. Just a final comment about gyms, if you join one that is more like a club do avoid the food which is often surprisingly fatty or sweet, and the alcoholic drinks.

Rehydrate with water not with wine, beer or sweet drinks. Also avoid the sports drinks and chocolate bars and take an apple to eat after exercising if you feel a little weak.

Yoga

A fantastic way to help your back as it is based on balance, stretching for flexibility (if you have a bad back you are usually stiff as a board) and strength (but not in a weight lifting sense). Men – don't be shy! Yes, you will be in the minority in the western world. Also don't worry that some people will be curling themselves up in knots when you are unable to reach your knees. The yoga teacher we had was absolutely great and said, "Peter, get as far as you can and then leave your imagination to do the rest." I think that was a lovely message because she was saying don't be too competitive with yourself. In yoga there is no competition between people you are aiming the best you can be with no pressure from others.

When I first went I could not touch my knees let alone my toes whilst some of the ladies could bend in two. I always felt very welcome and never intimidated only encouraged. Details can be found in local papers, sports halls or the local library. Word of mouth is always a good way to find good teachers. There are also yoga centres and associations that certify teachers and these will be a good source of information too.

Tai chi

A graceful sport that will build flexibility and some strength. There are many Tai Chi classes about run by people who are committed to the activity so details should be easy to find in local papers, sports halls or the local library.

Rowing/canoeing

Canoeing is good because it creates upper body strength and uses both sides of the body. Rowing is also good for the same reason but only if you have two oars (sculling). Pure rowing where you only have one oar is not good as it biases one side of your body. So leave that until you are recovered. Typically at a rowing club there will be an expectation that you also 'work out' so be minded of this – they may not have personal trainers who know anything about back problems. Their goal is usually to get people fit enough to win races – an extreme view I know, but based on experience.

Tennis, badminton and golf

These are all great sports both physically and socially. My recommendation though is to avoid these sports until your back is well on the mend as they bias one side of your body, which could set you back with a full recovery. Look at a tennis player serving and playing and you will instantly see what I mean. All I am saying is not yet, not, not ever.

ACTION

- What sports or exercises could you consider starting?

Chapter 6 – Remaining active and even taking up a new sport

- Find out where you can partake and when you can start.

- When could you start to walk, or increase the amount you are doing if you currently walk a little?

- Make plans to start to do something – and keep a log.

- Review progress.

Chapter 7

An easy way to flexibility

I have found one of the best ways to help solve a back problem is to increase your level of flexibility. Initially when your back is in spasm you may be as stiff as a board, in considerable pain and unable to bend at all, so the thought of any form of flexibility can at this stage, appear to be just a pipe dream.

No matter how little movement you have some basic stretching exercises will pay dividends. I have identified below a series of simple stretching exercises that you can do at any time and in any place.

> *NOTE: Always consult your medical practitioner before undertaking any exercises.* Act responsibly and if excessive pain or strain is experienced in attempting any of the actions explained in this book or if anyone is under medical supervision, it is recommended that they follow the advice of their doctor, medical practitioner or physiotherapist.

Stretch 1

Stand as upright as you can, feet about 30 centimetres apart (12 inches), and place your hands, palm down on the top of your thighs. Slowly lean forward and slide your hands down your thighs. Go as low as you can until you feel the stretch, maintaining some support with your hands. Hold for 30 seconds, or less if it is uncomfortable. Slowly stand back upright. If you are as stiff as a board you may only just move from vertical – that is fine, you are finding the point that you feel the stretch. Breathe normally.

Stretch 2

Stand as upright as you can, feet about 30 centimetres apart (12 inches), and place your hands on your lower back just above your hips. Palms to back, fingertips just touching on your spine and thumbs pointing down your outer waist. Slowly lean backwards until you feel the stretch, maintaining support with your hands and don't topple over. Hold for 30 seconds, or less if it is uncomfortable. Slowly stand back upright. Breathe normally.

Stretch 3

Stand as upright as you can, feet about 30 centimetres apart (12 inches), and about 30 centimetres from a table or kitchen work surface. Place your hands, palm down on the surface. Slowly lean forward supporting your weight on your hands. Go as low as you can until you feel the stretch in the back of your legs, maintaining support with your hands. Hold for 30 seconds, or less if it is uncomfortable. Slowly stand back upright. If you are as stiff as a board you may only just move from vertical – that is fine, you are finding the point that you feel the stretch. Breathe normally.

Next.

Whilst in this position take up the same stance and before you lean forward put your left foot back 30 centimetres (12 inches), keeping the left leg straight whilst slightly bending at the knee with the right leg. Now follow the previous instructions. Repeat with the right leg back and the left knee bent.

Stretch 4

Stand upright with your feet about 45 centimetres apart (18 inches). Reach up to the ceiling with your left hand and arm straight. Now bend at the elbow bringing your hand down, palm open behind your head so your hand rests on your upper back just to the right hand of the spine, and your thumb stretching over your spine. Fingers should be pointing down your back. Stand tall and feel the stretch. You may want to brace or hold yourself firm by holding a door frame with your right hand. Hold for 30 seconds, or less if it is uncomfortable. Breathe normally. Repeat with the right hand over your head.

Stretch 5

Stand as upright as you can, feet about 30 centimetres apart (12 inches). Hold a solid surface such as a worktop or door frame with your right hand. If you can, aim to bring your left foot up behind you and clasp it with your left hand. You will now be standing on just your right leg. Gently pull your foot up with your left hand until you feel a stretch in your thigh. Hold for 30 seconds, or less if it is uncomfortable. Slowly lower foot to the floor and stand upright. Breathe normally. Repeat with the right leg.

More advanced stretches are useful but these are enough to start you off. Never strain, it is always better to do just a little rather than over do it and set yourself back. The only person you are competing with is yourself. Don't forget to breathe though!

Never over-stretch or push yourself too hard. Also never 'bounce' to get the stretch working better, you will damage yourself and set yourself back. You have been warned.

Yoga

It would be valuable if you considered undertaking some yoga. This is not some cranky system to make you look silly or feel awkward but a way of increasing your flexibility. It may seem daft at the early stages of a major back problem but once you are able to move around a little I consider it to be a very valuable investment in time. Clearly in the early stages there is no way that you will be able to stretch and do positions anywhere near those of regular yoga class goers. Do not be deterred though. I have found that people are very understanding and considerate and are so keen to see you improve. Whilst your attempts look pathetic compared with other people in the yoga class it does not matter. In yoga the only person you are comparing yourself with, is in fact yourself. If you do not want to go to a yoga class I would suggest investing in a book on yoga or a DVD that shows you exercises to do.

When I went to yoga classes I could barely stand, I had no flexibility and it hurt to sit on the mat. This did not deter me and whilst some of the ladies were quite literally putting their feet behind their heads I couldn't even sit upright on the floor, as my back was so stiff. Help, encouragement and spending 90 minutes just focussing on me was hugely beneficial. I was also the only man in the group of 20 and initially I felt a little self-conscious although that soon eased as I was always made to feel so welcome. There is always a mixed standard in any group and at times it was great for some of the others to laugh with me at my attempts – over time I improved and we all celebrated in our successes.

I have also included yoga in the sports section for good reason too.

Frequency

I suggest that stretching exercises should be undertaken twice per day but do use other opportunities in the day to stretch a little.
It is always much better to do a little and often rather than a lot and not very often. You are teaching your body to be flexible and the only way is through a constant awareness that it takes small steps that build to create the overall change.

Other opportunities

An example of other opportunities for stretching would include when you are in the shower or bath, use the warmth of the water to relax tense muscles and put a gentle stretch into your body as part of your washing regime. These do not need to be intensive sessions of stretching, and do be careful not to slip. But do use this as an opportunity to do something.

Another good example would be to do a little stretching while you are waiting for the kettle to heat, the toast to pop up, an egg to boil. Many small stretches can be introduced into your normal routine, whilst watching television, reading, opening the post or doing pretty much any daily activity.

Simply sitting at the table gives you the opportunity to do some simple stretching exercises. For example, sit on the edge of your seat and stretch out one leg straight and rest it on the heel of your foot. You will instantly feel a tension in the back of your leg now gently lean your torso forward to increase the stretch. Hold for 30 seconds and then repeat with the other leg.

Another simple stretch that is easily done is to sit up straight rather than in a slight slouch that most people adopt and then stretch out your spine by easing your lower back forward. Hold for a few seconds and then relax and repeat. The range of stretches that you can introduce is large so have a little experimentation with this.

ACTION

- Start your stretching regime – slowly.

- Keep a daily schedule and record when you did your stretching.

- Record each stretch you do and the progress you are making.

- What else could you do to help your flexibility with your daily tasks?

Chapter 8

Posture: Looking and feeling good

Good posture is crucial for good back health.

People talk about the importance of having good posture but if you look at people in daily life most have anything but. The reason good posture is important is because it aligns all of your muscles and bones in a way that nature intended.

Quite simply if you are not looking after your posture it will cause you problems. If you don't continue to look after the way you walk, sit, stand you will continue to have problems. Some temporary, some that will become permanent.

It is critical to think about your posture in a conscious way for as much time as possible until good posture starts to become second nature. Consider, are you sitting in a chair reading this and are you slumped right now?

When walking you should think about the way you 'carry' yourself. Are you walking with rounded shoulders and head hung low? Are you holding your back straight and trying to pull in the lower part of your back so you stand erect? Are you holding in your tummy? Are your shoulders back and chin forward? Or are you just not bothering about how your walk and stand?

The key thing about maintaining good quality back care is actually ensuring that you stand or sit with good posture. The important thing is to understand what is the right posture for you. So firstly, when you're in perfect health, if you stand upright you should have an inward curve in the lower part of your back, it's called the lordosis, and that should be there naturally with your tummy nicely pulled in, shoulders back, and head back. If you look at most people walking around, sitting or going about their daily life, there's not that many people who actually carry themselves very well. I'm not saying everyone should have a military posture where you hold a real stiff stance but make sure that you're being kind to your body by maintaining the best shape possible and the shape you would ideally like it to be. The shape nature intended.

An extremely useful way to develop your own good posture is to start taking note of how other people sit, stand and walk – become an observer. This is a hugely valuable opportunity so that you can start to get an excellent idea of what good posture is, and importantly what it is not. Now compare what you have seen and witnessed with other people and how you deport yourself? When you pass a shop window look at your own reflection. Are you standing or walking well? Stop yourself in your mental tracks when you are sitting and consider if you are sitting well or have fallen into bad habits.

So review:

- When you sit in a car do you have a good posture?
- What about sitting at the table, when you're eating or reading a paper?
- What about sitting at your desk?
- How well do you sit on a sofa?
- When you're walking.
- The various places that you will be during the course of the day.
- How do you walk up stairs?
- How do you carry your bags?

Take each one and ask:

- Am I standing correctly, correctly for me? Have I got that lower curve at the base of my spine?

- Does my tummy stick out too much and if so is that because my posture is not very good, or perhaps, I'm carrying just a bit too much weight?
- Are my shoulders nicely back, have I got gently sloping shoulders, is my head back?
- Or am I stooped and leaning forward and carrying the weight of the world across my shoulders, as so many people seem to? If you are, it's putting an enormous pressure on your back by not standing correctly.
- How are your feet positioned?
- Are your knees bent or straight?
- Are you standing so one leg is taking all of your weight?
- Are you standing with your hips level or with one knee bent and the other leg straight?

All of these things will have an impact.

My whole objective with this book is to help you to live a natural life, to live a life where your posture is good, and where it doesn't matter if at times it's not. That you can actually sit in an uncomfortable chair and it won't matter, for a while. Where you are generally taking care of yourself and your way of living is being back-aware at a less conscious level.

Walking

Think about when you're walking how do you walk, do you shuffle or do you walk quite smartly? Are you carrying things only in one hand so, for example, a very heavy briefcase or bag in one hand and nothing in the other? This possibly means that you are twisting yourself. Is that good for your posture? If you have to carry one bag that is heavy, is it better to periodically switch it from side to side. I know if it's very heavy there would be a natural tendency to do that anyway. If you have a dominant hand either left handed or right handed, there will be a tendency to put a handbag, a shopping bag, a briefcase, a tool bag or whatever it is, just in one hand as you walk along. If it's not too heavy the tendency is to leave it just in the one dominant hand. Now just think, if it's heavy but not too heavy are you causing damage by constantly causing a twist and strain on one side of your body?

Sitting in a car

When sitting in a car, is the car seat heavily reclined? Or is it too bolt upright? Is it too close to the steering wheel or is it too far away so you have to stretch? Are you sitting stooped as many people do? Look around you at the traffic lights when you're in a car. How are people sitting and do you think that they have good posture or not? Look at other people, whether on the bus, on the train or even an aeroplane. How are they sitting, how are you sitting, which is the best way? Are you sitting upright enough but with a little recline, just to take the pressure off your lower back? Become aware.

Sitting at a table

I would always advocate eating your main meals at a table sitting in a dining chair. Sitting in front of the television, with your lunch or dinner on a tray, stooped over trying to eat is no good for your digestion and certainly is appalling for your posture. If you do this as a family, just look at the shape of everyone else. Their mind is on what is happening on television without any consideration for their bodies. Now ask yourself 'what back problems are they storing up for later in life?' Use a table. Sit upright, eat correctly, and allow digestion to take place properly. When at a table everything can be at your fingertips as well. Certainly if you are in a lot of pain, the one place you do not want to be sitting is that "comfortable" sofa in front of the television. You need to be sitting at a table so you can brace yourself if needed when in pain. This also encourages your body to align itself properly.

Sitting on an easy chair or sofa

When sitting in an easy chair or sofa consider how you are sitting.

- Are you all curled up in a ball?
- Are you hunched up?
- Is it so soft and cosy that you are making your back worse?
- Or is it one which is an excellent shape, supportive where it needs to be, is allowing you to sit with great posture where your knees aren't around your ears?
- Are your feet flat on the floor?
- If you want to curl up in a ball or stretch out on the sofa – is it wise?
- Is there sufficient support around you, and by using occasional cushions in the right place can you provide greater support?
- Do you get so absorbed in a film on television that you lose concentration of how you are sitting only to regret it at a later time? So critically, review how you are sitting, wherever you happen to be it will be worth it!

In the early stages of getting yourself well again when you have major back problems you will feel uncomfortable anywhere. So you may as well get into good habits at this point by consciously sitting in the right type of chair, and aiming to sit in a good position. There's a chapter elsewhere in this book that provides a brief guide on the type of furniture to use. This way you can start to educate yourself about the best posture and learn to take care of yourself.

I would add that once you have learnt to sit properly you will find it much easier if confronted with an uncomfortable chair to find a way of getting properly comfortable that won't damage your back again. Alternatively your tolerance will be much lower and you will find a better chair to sit on.

Some simple tips when sitting

These are just a few thoughts to help your posture:

- Avoid squashy unsupportive seats.
- Do not to sit on anything too low – to get out of the seat you will put enormous strain on your back. Observe how others manage.
- Aim to sit in a chair with arms so they will give you firm support to rise from the seat.
- Don't sit for too long. I suggest getting up every 20 minutes, if only for a brief stretch.
- Aim to have a chair where there is support for your whole spine, or your lower back at least.
- Keep both feet flat on the floor.
- Ideally your knees should be slightly lower than your hips if you are sitting at a desk or table.
- Do 'wriggle' and keep your spine supported.
- Put a cushion in your lower back – and try and lean back, only then pad any other gaps with a cushion.
- Interestingly, old fashioned furniture is usually better designed than modern furniture.
- Tired 20 year old sofas that were once modern looking are usually a disaster to sit in.
- If grandma struggles to sit in it and falls the last few inches and says, 'ooo that's better' avoid the seat like the plague.
- If your grandma struggles to get out of it, it probably is not a good seat to sit in. Grandma certainly does know best!
- Do not feel obliged to sit on the one chair that you are directed to.
- If visiting people and your back is painful ask for a dining chair to sit on.
- A hot water bottle can be wonderful to relax tense muscles – just make sure it does not leak!

I am sure with trial and hopefully few errors you will add to the list.

When I was out and offered a seat that I thought unsuitable I used to say, I'd love to sit there, and thank you, but have you got a dining room chair I can sit on? I no longer have a problem sitting pretty much anywhere but if I am likely to be seated for some time and the offered seat does look a little 'too comfortable and soft' I still ask for an alternative. No one takes offence.

Posture aids

This is an interesting area and one where there is a whole industry ready to provide anything that you could think of and many things that you probably can't.

I started using some aids to help me walk and get back into shape when I was in the process of recovering and I soon realised what was happening. I started to become dependent on them. Interesting, or frightening? I soon stopped using them, and have not used them since and this was because I could easily see I would be holding back my recovery.

There are a lot of devices out on the market place and if you go to the last few pages of many magazines or newspapers it's not unusual to find adverts suggesting a whole range of products such as:

- Foam rolls for your back.
- Massage machines.
- Wooden ball seat covers.
- Special seats to carry around with you.
- Foam wedges.
- Elastic corsets.
- Special braces for your back.
- Vests with metal bars in them to support your spine.
- The list goes on....

I am not saying there is no place for these products but I found that it is so easy to keep buying items thinking that they are the one thing that will make the difference. In my case they did not and I wasted a serious amount of money. I also had illusions of quick cures and those never happened either, with the resulting disappointment.

Anything elasticised that goes around your body, especially if it has reinforcing ribs in it means that you will start to loose muscle strength around the very area where you need to be strong. If you walk with a frame or a stick you will start to become dependent upon it. If you start to use special seats, what happens when you go somewhere where there isn't one, or you forget yours? At worst you start to become a prisoner in your own home.

When you walk past cars parked with the disabled badge you will see a fairly motley looking selection of foam rolls and supports on the seats. They are using a device to solve a problem and unless they have one in their bag as well they probably have difficulty when out and about. To me this is self-defeating, so if the car seat is appalling do something about it. If it's not, try to get used to using what is available and by changing your posture, by flexing your muscles a little bit. By keeping yourself in good shape your body will adapt to different situations and you will not have problems.

All the aids I have found have been totally self-defeating and not the focus of this book. I want you to live normal life.

One's lower spine should gently curve inwards. When my back 'went' it bulged outwards quite alarmingly. I was a mess so when I sat down I just could not get comfortable anywhere. I tried some of the foam rolls but found that things I had around the house worked for me. A folded clean towel. A cushion from the sofa. A pillow to sit on.

In reality these worked better. A pillow folded in two and placed on a seat with the folded part at the back meant that there was a gentle forward slope, which was perfect. It raised the seat too so it was much easier to get out of. The folded towel could be adjusted and the ends that popped out either side made it easier to move about. These are also things other people have in their homes so if you are out visiting friends they can easily help while you are recovering.

By the way, if you do use pillows and towels make sure it is for the short term so set a review deadline – in your diary or on the calendar. And keep them clean, respect yourself and your home.

You don't need to spend money to have things that will help with your posture. If your old sofa is not right for you, somewhere in your home you will have a dining chair, kitchen chair or chair in one of the bedrooms that will do just fine. Sometimes even a garden chair is a better shape – clean it up, bring it in the house!

Final comment

Do take some time to consider your posture. You may have had years of being quite happy with the way you walk, sit or stand. If you have a back problem there is the probability that some aspect of your posture is not right. Now is a great time to start to 'retrain' the way you go about your daily routines.

Once you have got used to thinking about your back health it will soon become a part of the way you live. You will look better, stand, sit and walk far better and it will be an integral part of keeping yourself in good shape. It will become natural and no one will take any notice of your past problem.
Just be careful of those squashy 'comfortable' chairs.

ACTION

- Start right now and review your posture – how are you sitting, how do you walk, how do you stand?

- How does your posture change when you sit in that 'comfortable' chair, in a car, when you eat?

- Be conscious about your posture as often as you can.

- Ask someone else to keep an eye on you and remind you when you could do better. Then thank them for their care, don't get irritated with them. You need to value their support.

- How frequently are you getting up to move about?

- Are you using posture aids that you could reduce your dependency on? If yes, what is your deadline for getting rid of them?

Chapter 9

Harnessing the power of the mind in recovery

A significant part ensuring a good and as speedy a recovery as possible is to combat concerns that your mind will keep raising. It is amazing how restricting one's mind can be in telling us that there are things that we cannot do. The pain associated with back problems can be overwhelming, however a key part in gaining mobility and a normal life is to master matters of the mind so that you can move forward. This may seem like fanciful thinking but do continue reading as this is a fundamental 'blockage' that separates most people who get better from those who do not.

It is fairly clear why this happens as our body has an automatic survival system built in that was developed as part of our early legacy as human beings. So early in fact that this part of the brain is called the 'mammalian brain', which is part of our overall brain. It is the part that runs our body systems on automatic pilot, such as breathing, immune system, beating of our heart and reflex actions. If we put our hand on something hot we automatically and quickly pull our hand away. This is what is happening with back problems too, but this part of the brain was formed 100,000s years ago and is not always providing us with the service we need and deserve. We are no longer cave dwellers and finding our food in a world where there were many predators, where we, and our predators, were running around the prairie or jungle.

This is not to say ignore what is going on but to work with the reaction in a conscious way rather than an unconscious way. Do not be frightened by this thought – it is your body and you need to be in control of what is happening.

Chapter 9 – Harnessing the power of the mind in recovery

It is easy to talk about having a positive attitude but this is critically important in gaining momentum in speeding your recovery.

A simple start is to provide a cheery voice to ourselves when we are preparing for the day. No negative talk, so focus on getting better rather than 'stewing in our own juice'.

When greeting people be positive, be keen, be warm and friendly. You know people who are negative, even if they are completely fit – it is very tiring being in their presence. So think of the impact you are having on those people who you see – if you are bright and positive it brings light into their day. It may mean that they are keen to spend time with you. Perhaps keen to help with the things you genuinely cannot do because they know they are not being used and will be appreciated.

I know only too well that it can be an utter misery and a real effort trying to be pleasant when all you want is to be quiet and alone. The key is to be positive for the short time that you are with people, but, and it is a vital but, do make it clear that when they visit or want to spend time with you that this is framed so there are clear limits and expectations.

It is far better to say to someone "I am struggling, would love to see you, but please accept that I need my own space so can the visit be, say 10 minutes?". It may be that if you share your home with others that they can then carry on the conversation in another room with other people. If a friend comes round every day at coffee time and it is not what you can cope with, say you would love to see them every other day, or what suits you best, and if the time needs to be different do say so too. The respectful way of seeing people is to make sure that you are 'present' with them and enjoy their company so when they leave they think that it was a good visit and will want to return. If you sit with a moaner who is miserable, no matter how much you love them you will find excuses to visit less often! Be warned.

You will be making time for your exercises and other activities so it should be expected that the time you have for entertaining will not be open ended. Also do not use the distraction of others to delay what you know needs to be done to speed your recovery.

Do remember the people around you, who are part of your support mechanism, need their own space and time too, or else they will get tired and make themselves ill. This may, at times, make you feel vulnerable or 'abandoned'. This is not the case and all too often people who are called upon to help ending up getting tired too. This will cause some factors that you had not expected. Even in the best relationships this can cause niggles and some irritability – often this is just because the other person is getting tired and possibly stressed too. This can also be because you are being too demanding and nothing ever seems good enough, or not the way you exactly want something done. You may be taking out your own frustrations on them.

I was always so grateful when people did something to help out, although you will have gathered I would try and do as much as possible, taking it all as part of my own rehabilitation. But on the occasions, when people did do something I would prefer that they didn't, I learnt that it can be wiser to just let some things go, and be thankful that there is help at hand. An example of what I mean is I like weak tea, no sugar. When you have had to drink your tea in the kitchen time and time again it is wonderful when someone says they will make it and bring it to – even if strong and with sugar in it!

One of the other ways people around you get irritable is when they see you doing nothing and being content to let others run around doing everything for you. I stress, and will mention this many times, do make the effort to do something. Also don't make a fuss over it and show how tough it is and then give up for a few more days. Your attitude is in your mind – it can be tough and horrible or a challenge you will get pleasure from mastering – the choice is yours, the task is the same. Persist – it does get better!

Positive Mental Attitude – or as it is sometimes called a PMA. I am keen on us all being positive, I am not keen on creating a positive mental attitude without action. Anyone can sit and be positive and do nothing and hope the world will change for them. This is utterly useless – as always, action is key.

Meditation

When you are wracked with pain this may seem totally daft. Well if you haven't tried it don't knock it! The simple act of consciously doing nothing is great – well I say do nothing, you are aiming to meditate. This can take many forms and if you are interested there are whole books written on various types. What I will cover here is only intended to whet your appetite and help you realise that this is something that you can add into your daily activity.

When you meditate you **do not** fall asleep, you go into a deep relaxed state where the purpose is to allow your mind to have space so it can regenerate.

The process is simple. Sit or kneel or lie down and relax – acknowledge your body and work down from head to toe tensing muscles and then relaxing and letting go of that part of the body. This will cause some discomfort but go with it (an added benefit is if you are very immobile it can at least give each of your muscles a little work out).

Typically this is what you do:

- Tighten your scalp, hold for 5 seconds and then slowly let go and relax.
- Now screw up your face hold for 5 seconds and slowly let go and relax.
- Tense your bite for 5 seconds and slowly let go and relax.
- Continue the same process with your arms, tummy muscles, leg muscles, feet, each time you will learn more

about your body and where there is tension and possibly pain.

- Once you have completed the tense/relax process just allow your body to relax completely and start to concentrate on nothing, if a thought comes to mind acknowledge it and let it go, then another thought may come, let it go too, don't give any thought power and slowly a peace of mind will arrive.

I have found once I have successfully relaxed and my mind goes still it is wonderful to find that inner peace even if only for a few moments. When you have reached this state it is important to enjoy the moment but don't stay there for too long – the whole process should only take about 20 - 30 minutes.

Once you have reached a quiet state, do start to focus your thoughts on the part of your back that is causing you pain – now really focus your mind on the specific area and tell yourself you are getting better.

Some may think this is mumbo jumbo, well isn't it worth a try? There is increasing evidence that if we can focus our minds on a specific part of the body and ailments it really can work. You are not doing anything else anyway – so it is worth a go?!! If the alternative is another TV show, I know where my money is. Aim to do this daily, some people suggest twice daily.

Tratak

In yoga there is a relaxation process called tratak. You can use a candle, which I prefer, in a darkened room, or you can use a flower in a lighter room. (If you are by yourself I do not recommend a candle due to the fire hazard in case you fall asleep or cannot get up to blow it out.) This is where you sit and go through the relaxation process of relaxing your body as if you are starting to meditate. The main difference is you use the candle or flower as the focus – the candle or flower being about 3 metres

(10feet) away. You are not really looking at the object just focussing your eyes on this point and then slowly relaxing your eyes so you don't focus at all.

The relaxing slowly allows you to acknowledge your body and get used to where specific aches and pains are rather than thinking generally.

One of the biggest problems I found was that suddenly you move from being an active member of society, to being completely debilitated. There is nothing going on that you have control of. The whole of your life closes down other than the very world that you see from either your bed or your armchair. This is supplemented by what other people may share with you, but that is it. This change can be so huge. In my case I went from health to non-health very rapidly and watching my life close down around me was horrifying.

There is a stage when you know there is no escape, in the short-term, from this back pain. You hope and think it may suddenly click back or something amazing will happen and all will be fine. But soon you realise that it's not going to happen and you have got to come to terms with things. This was a big issue for me. I'd been very active sports wise, very active in business and hugely active from a social point of view. I'd had a very full life and suddenly almost everything stopped. Getting my mind around that was massively important from a sanity point of view and from a recovery point of view too.

Getting your mind around things is hugely important.

I've mentioned the use of medication in one of the other chapters of this book – some people use it to still the mind, some to get to sleep – my recommendation is to avoid any medication unless there is a very sound reason. And this is a reason you have challenged yourself about and also challenged your medical practitioner about too.

If, and this should be a BIG 'IF' you take medication ask the crucial question – what date do you intend to stop taking the medication? This is a big ask of yourself and your situation and I cannot stress enough how important this one question is.

> **Note:**
> The answer to this question is so important as it indicates the state of your mind and the attitude you have towards your problem. Do you see it as a short term problem you are going to deal with or submit to the excuse that this is a long term problem? You have a choice.

I found that I had a lot of negative self-talk. Things going through my mind such as:

- I have got major problems
- I can't go to work
- I won't be able to feed myself properly
- It was a major trip to the loo and painful
- I can't drive at all
- I can't walk
- .....and many other things telling me everything I could not do.

I found this quite destructive and very unsettling so I decided to 'reframe' my life. Instead of focussing on what I could not do, I made a decision, no matter how tough things got to focus on what I **could** do.

This was a major step.

It meant that I was taking responsibility. I started to acknowledge and get excitement from very small things that started to become a part of my journey to get back on my feet and getting back to normality.

I needed to lower my expectations from where they were before and not get annoyed or down beat if I failed to achieve what I had managed when I was fit. This is easier said than done but crucial to set the new 'start point'.

One of the things that I also completed was a diary so I could see what I had achieved. At times it made depressing reading but if I had a poor day I made sure that the following day would be better, even if only by one small thing. That one small thing could then be celebrated often with a smile of self satisfaction. (When you read the part on eating, you will realise that a large cream cake as celebration is a counterproductive reward!)

If there is no measurement kept and poor standards are set then life will not be centred on achievement, only on an acceptance of mediocrity. It is surprising how quickly some people will give up and accept the status quo. This may sound cruel or even smug – it is a sad reality. If you have slipped back take responsibility and start to think and do things differently – and the best time to start is RIGHT NOW. There is nothing in your way other than yourself……is there?

Set small goals and reset when they are achieved. The mind is a powerful tool – used positively it is amazing what it will help us do. The same is true if we don't use it!

One hears of people who set huge goals, strive to achieve them and then make them – they all do it one step at a time. So if you have set a huge goal you will need to set small steps on the journey to it. If you try and get there in one leap it is not realistic. You know that – your mind knows that and will not be fooled. The answer to the question 'How do you eat an elephant?' is always the same 'one bite at a time'. Getting fit again and returning to good health will be one step at a time too.

Lowering expectations was never part of my life. I'd always be quite competitive, in the world of business and the world of sport. I enjoyed a very busy social life as well. The thought of saying 'I

am not going to do those things' or 'I **cannot** do those things' – two very different sets of words I hasten to add, was a huge realisation. The 'can't do' was the shock of knowing what I could do before my back problem and after. No matter how bad things are we have choices – I could think 'doom, gloom, despondency, life has stopped'. I felt that life was on hold and I needed to do something. Lowering expectations was horrible but it gave me a realistic base to start from.

The expectation that I could go to work for a ten hour day, plus drive an hour each way, was totally unrealistic. I could mentally conceive it but my body would not allow it. I reached the stage where I thought I was in a horrible place. My mind seemed to want to take over and the fears of incapability, and worse, started to lock me in a mental prison. This is where I thought I needed some small 'wins' to boost my esteem. At this time almost anything was a small win. So, by lowering my expectation I had not removed all of my expectations, just set a much, much lower bar to jump over. A bar I set realistically so I could achieve some 'wins'.

When we hear of someone in public life who has had an illness or major injury we are delighted when they start to regain full health. We almost celebrate each small step and this is what we have to do ourselves.

It's like a footballer who used to play a full 90 minutes on the pitch. Often, when they return to playing after an injury, they play only for a short period of time, sometimes as little as five or ten minutes. This does not imply they are no good. It's just part of their rehabilitation. They are back on the field for a short period of time to see how they get on in a competitive situation with the full crowd and audience pressure. The match performance is very different from being on a training ground having a practice kick around. A training match does not emulate the real full professional game. I lowered my expectation levels to a point where I believed I could make the most of myself. I did not set unachievable targets otherwise I would have a day full of underachievement – something that is not good for the spirit!

Act like the professional player determined to perform well for 10 minutes and be pleased with your progress. Not the sulking amateur.

This **is** a mindset issue – we could say of the sports person playing 10 minutes of a game 'isn't it pathetic they have only managed to be on the sports field for 10 minutes' OR 'isn't it great that they have managed 10 minutes and are getting back into the game' – a mindset shift is needed from one to the other. Treat yourself with respect and celebrate the achievement.

One of the challenges I set myself was to make a cup of tea. Simple under 'normal' circumstances. These were not normal circumstances. This was a challenge to rise to. One where the elements of making the tea needed to be broken down into small steps. Each step an achievement when completed. Each step combining to make the complete challenge. So the steps in outline were and still are:

- Get to the kitchen
- Put a kettle on
- Make a cup of tea
- Get cup of tea back to chair to drink
- Drink the cup of tea.

I have made the sub tasks quite large, you can imagine that the 'Make a cup of tea' stage is also broken down into steps such as:

- Get cup and saucer out of cupboard
- Get teaspoon out
- Get teapot out
- Get tea out of a different cupboard
- Get milk out of fridge

Each step is a challenge, each step is a composite part of the whole. When you achieve something that was difficult, or impossible before, it should be celebrated. It is a step on the road to recovery.

How easy it is when there are other people about to let them wait on you! Don't!

Initially I would get a small bottle of water, partially filled, put it in my pocket and get back to the chair where I would drink it. I could have stayed at this level but I made the decision that I no longer wanted cold water all the time. It was winter and a hot drink was what I wanted. Making a cup of tea and drinking it in the kitchen perched on a stool was a huge success, when I managed to get the cup back to my sitting room you can imagine the pride. I can still feel it now! I was getting better. I was getting my mind in shape. I had raised my 'bar'.

This is where the mind shift happens at a personal level and the education of those who support you. *I cannot stress this area too much – this is really where rehabilitation starts.*

It is not the cup of tea. It is the start of taking responsibility and your intention to get better. If you can do it for one cup of tea you can do it for everything.

Visualisation

One of my loves in life is walking on the hills and I missed not being able to just get up and go. So what I did was start to visualise me walking on the hills I know and enjoy. I placed myself as a fit person striding out and standing and staring at the view. I imagined being out on the hills on a cold crisp winter day. On a warm fresh spring day. Kicking the leaves on a dry autumn day. That became a goal to aim for. A goal that I could really imagine with all of my senses. Have you a goal that you really want to achieve?

Chapter 9 – Harnessing the power of the mind in recovery

So I started to work out what I would need to do to make what I pictured a reality. Thinking about walking on the hills again was a mind step so far adrift from where I was but it provided a focus for the longer term. Something to aim for and something that raised valuable questions such as:

- What are the small steps I needed to take to get going?
- How will I measure my development?
- How could I get started?
- What did I need to do right now?
- What could I do first?

I had to start somewhere so starting the journey to the kitchen was my first target – it was one I was going to make several times a day so I could measure my results and see what changes I could make. It initially took 20 minutes. Just the simple task of measuring and recording the times gave me a focus and a goal. It also gave me a measure too. I could start to see the changes, second by second and then minutes by minute. Yes, there were times when it took longer than the last, which at the time could have been quite demoralising but taking a longer view it was clear progress was being made, albeit not linear.

The very nature of looking for improvements meant that I no longer accepted things as they were. This was another big turning point, and will be a big turning point for you too.

Ask yourself 'Am I making a difference?' Do not accept the fact it might take 10 minutes to complete a task and fail to look for any improvement. If it took 10 minutes when I first timed it that was my starting benchmark so the next time I would set a new target time that was a stretch but not ridiculous. So I would take it down in seconds – let's do it in 9 minutes and 50 seconds, 9 minutes 40. So each step was sufficiently small enough not to be a failure but sufficiently large enough to be a challenge. And in this example it may be that I would set a target for the day rather than change it for every journey. Think, if you had only reduced the target by 10 seconds a day, within a week that is over a minute and within a month the time would be halved to just 4 minutes 50 seconds. Now that would be progress I am sure you agree. And each day you can celebrate those achievements.

So what target are you going to set?

With many illnesses there is an expected timescale for recovery. With back problems it is rare for there to be a specific time for recovery. This can play havoc with one's mind. Many of us want to get better quickly albeit I've seen people who, realising that they can't get better quickly, don't choose to get better at all. Odd, but true.

I worked on the principle that each day I would make some noticeable difference somewhere to make sure I was on that journey of recovery. My general practitioner, who was excellent, was unable to give me a time span for recovery. Some people said I'd never recover – for me that wasn't an option. The neurosurgeon I was under (to reaffirm again I have not had surgery) was talking about months so I set my target as months. Months to me meant a few months not many months. A mindset choice.

That was my time span. Ultimately the timeframe is down to you – how much you do, how many steps you take on the journey, how hard you push yourself, how hard you are on yourself to make things better. It is easy to set very high challenges and push yourself too hard. You may try to stretch too hard and cause a bigger problem. You may set the bar too high and fail to clear it, and I deliberately use the word fail, as you may start to become despondent and think this is no good, it's useless, there's no point in carrying on because every time I set a challenge, I fail.

BUT if you set it too low it becomes so easy that you think that was not worth the bother, so it's a balance point. The only person who can tell you where the challenge point is, is yourself.

I mentioned my journey to the kitchen as an example. You may find the following day it takes longer than it did originally because you pushed yourself. Don't lose heart – sometimes the extra challenge is just what you need so you can really dig deep and move forward. Sometimes it is just a little too much. Time and trying will tell you what the answer is. It is always better to keep the challenge there rather than be too soft and easy.

ACTION

- Start each day with a cheerful thought. Greet people with an upbeat attitude.

- Are you considering the people around you and making sure that they have their space and time and you are not overburdening them?

- Start to take time to focus on your body in a still way through meditation or simple relaxation.

- If you are on medication when do you intend to stop – what date? You need to take responsibility for this and discuss with your medical practitioner.

- Start to keep a log so you know what is happening and you can look at progress.

- What are your goals and what is the first step you are going to take?

- Celebrate small wins rather than be defeatist with small setbacks.

- What goal can you start to visualise that you wish to achieve? Now work out the steps to make this reality.

Chapter 10

Managing and working through stress

Stress can be a major contributory cause of back problems. Stress is also something that will ensure back problems continue longer than they should. It is important when you have a back problem to aim to reduce the levels of stress in your life as much as possible. When in a state of stress problems can be caused in your body because of the tension in muscles, which you will feel as a spasm and creates hard feeling muscles. This causes your spine to become even more twisted and increase the pain that you are suffering.

In Chapter 1 it was mentioned that the fear associated with a back problem can be quite profound. This fear in itself will cause stress. This stress will delay your recovery. So as tough and as counter intuitive this may sound you need to relax to allow the healing to take place as quickly as possible.

I found that the more I worried and became anxious about my pain the slower I was to start to take action. Action to start my recovery.

The very fact that you are in such significant pain will make you feel stressed. You will be stressed about areas such as:

- The way you feel physically.
- The impact it's having on life.
- The impact it is having on your work.
- Stressed about 'when can I get back to work?'
- The impact on your income.

- The impact that will have both on you and your family members you have at home.
- Your social life.
- Promises that you have made to others that you cannot fulfil.

The list goes on.

The pressure builds up and everything associated with the debility you now have magnifies itself.

I found at a personal level things started to get out of proportion and I became tense and edgy with myself and with others. I wanted to move forward, I was trying to push myself as much as possible but in a way which wasn't very well informed. I snapped at people around me, went off my food and the overall impact was significant – my physical and mental approach to the whole problem was wrong.

People who suffer with stress are often the first people to deny that they're experiencing stress.

After being so active to suddenly become totally inactive was a major challenge. My whole body was in tension as I was holding myself rigid to protect myself, to try and avoid any more pain. I found this extreme, from well being to immobility, very stressful at a physical level as I could do so little as anything I did do hurt.

From a mental point of view I was aware that everything in my life had stopped. And stopped suddenly. This was an important lesson I had to learn – that I could no longer do what I had taken for granted and needed to have a change of mindset. Everything I enjoyed doing was now denied me – life had suddenly hit rock bottom. If this has happened to you I know you understand. The key point here is to know that things will get better and it is up to you to reframe your life and make that decision.

I started to realise that sometimes I just could not move, I had got stuck through the stress and made my body so rigid that I was frightened to move. What I did was relax a little so I could start to move and decide to go and do a small job, to do anything to change my mindset. It could have been going to the kitchen and completing some preparation for the next meal, or make a drink. Just something to break the cycle. The sheer exhaustion of doing anything was a strain so once I had settled back I had a sense of achievement. It **is** important to realise that you have achieved something – even though, when compared with when you are fit, it is small. It is an achievement so acknowledge it. When you do something even larger celebrate it with a smile and then relax. Try and relax in a way which would ease both your body and your mind.

I developed ways of doing things. I would start to control my breathing, stop panting and being stressed by taking much deeper breaths. Sometimes this was physically painful because my rib cage expanded, which impacted upon my back and therefore the pain levels rose. I slowly took deeper breaths and by slowing down the pace little by little I found I could start to manage much better. Often I would do this if I became very stressed and in a lot of pain. I would also do this prior to getting up, either from bed in the morning or when I needed to get out of the chair I sat in.

It is important to acknowledge at times you may not be able to go to work. You may be holding up your family and people who are part of your life. You may be unable to go out and enjoy events that you could before. What you can do though is to determine what you are able to do while you have limited mobility. Decide to use the time productively and do something valuable – invest in yourself and your future. While you are doing this other people in your life can go out and do the things they would like to. If you restrict them, at worst you will be resented.

In the early stages of my recovery I started to read anything as a form of distraction. I could only manage light articles and magazines because my level of pain was high. Also to hold a book was a very difficult challenge. I then moved to novels, which had a decent plot so I could get caught up in the story, and let my mind become absorbed in a different world from my own. That was great because it took me away from my discomfort, the pain and also the fact that I wasn't an active person. I found that hugely valuable. I also started to realise that I was managing to have some time where I was not aware of constant pain. This was another major step forward as I realised my mind was capable of switching off the pain. Do you read anything that could be a good distraction?

After a while I got tired of some of the novels and, because my illness was quite prolonged, I started to read better quality books, ones with more interest, something that was valuable from a lifestyle point of view. An example was looking at bird books, which do interest me. This led me onto looking at a book about walking and thinking about getting back on the hills, and because I would understand the area better I would get more pleasure. I would also know what type of birds to expect to see. I also love maps so I started to see what route I could take by finding simple low level walks with few obstacles. This started to get me enthusiastic to get better and get out enjoying nature and the countryside. Whilst this was a not going to happen quickly it gave me something to aim for. Life started to look up because I was researching things that I wanted to do when I knew (and I do use the word strongly – *knew*) that I'd be back on my feet! What interests are you developing or revisiting?

One of the positive aspects of my illness was my speed of reading improved enormously, which was very useful. I was not a slow reader anyway so this added bonus was going to be useful back at work. It is important to celebrate these benefits, even though they may be hard won!

For some it's easy to sit and say 'no I can't do anything' and just get stressed about it. I recommend it is far better to take responsibility and look to a great future and prepare for it.

Initially it was like my life had crashed into a brick wall and I suddenly realised that I was not going to get out of the wreckage very quickly. It was a very tough period but the way I got through this phase was to acknowledge what I could still do, and do it. That shows that things are still possible. Even if they are small things it is wise to celebrate and build from them. The worst thing to do is to stop and do nothing. Anything you can do will start to restore some faith, some confidence.

I know I felt very sorry for myself and felt stressed out about the whole situation I found myself in. I asked "what small thing can I do which will give me a feeling that I'm making some progress, no matter how small it is". There is always something – what is it for you?

You know the old Chinese proverb that "A journey of a thousand leagues starts with one step". Well, I chose to take one step, even though it's a very small step, because then it means that the journey is just that little bit shorter.

Music

Most of us have music systems of some sort that are operated by a remote control handset. It is a great way to relax by having some restful music available to play. You may love rap music – I am not sure if it is the most conducive for relaxation though! I used some very restful music that I enjoyed and could drift away whilst I sat. I could feel the stress levels ebb away. Do use music just to chill out by, to relax and take the tempo of life down a little bit.

What music do you enjoy and find relaxing? Are you listening to it?

Medication

The temptation is to think that medication is needed for stress. I fought that tooth and nail to avoid taking any pills and potions. Life does not get better with medication as a general rule – it should only ever be a stop gap. You become dependent upon it, you want the tablets but they can become habit forming. I have met people who have been on some medication for years. I fortunately managed to avoid this and I would certainly encourage anyone who is in a similar situation to me to use medication ONLY as a last resort after detailed discussion with a doctor. If you start to take medication on a regular basis challenge this – you need to be in control of yourself, with some medication you will lose your 'edge'. Always remember that it is your responsibility to manage what medication you take – once a doctor has prescribed for you and you have left the consulting room they are onto the next patient and will not have time to keep reflecting on your circumstances.

Meditation

Another method I used was trying meditation. I am sure some people will think this is a bit odd when you are immobile and in pain. My view was I wasn't going anywhere anyway so why not try! Concentrate on something which is important for you, and let your mind go – so you aim to empty it of all thoughts, so you allow space that other wonderful things in life will start to fill. I remember a wonderful approach to anything, that "A thought is only a thought unless you give it power." Wonderful. The pain is a thought and you can train yourself not to give it power. You can train your mind to release the stress too – for what is stress, just worry. If you can relax, stop worrying and start to think of the next step, much of your stress will ebb away. Try it – you may find it works for you.

Meditation works very well listening to music that has a pleasant meaning for you. The music can take you to good places but it needs to be soothing and not too loud. I like classical music, and to anybody who says they don't like classical music, just hunt around a bit and you will find something that works for you. I would imagine I was in the concert hall sitting in the best seat right in the centre listening to the orchestra play, feeling the vibrations of the music sensing the mood of the audience, the skill of the players. Noticing when the tempo changed, when the music went quieter and when it started to become louder, the delicate pauses and the direction each instrument was playing from. In time I would relax and the pain would ease as the stress eased. It may work for you so try it.

You also have to think in a way that perhaps we wouldn't normally think. You have to be able to open your mind to doing new things and trying new things to help to relieve the stress. Because it's easy to fall back into the rut. As Earl Nightingale learnedly said back in the 50s "A rut is a grave with the ends kicked out." I had no intention of being in a rut, so it is genuinely thinking about what you can do so that you feel that you are achieving something. It is better to do something than nothing even if that something is nowhere near as much as you were achieving before. Those small things all add up and will eventually start to become larger successes. I found each and every thing I did became little stress-busters, which meant that the ability to put a more positive face to the world became far easier.

Flexibility

Moving on to a slightly different issue – flexibility. I know this is covered elsewhere but it is important to make a few extra points here. When you've got back problems sometimes it's very difficult to maintain your whole body flexibility. When my back went, which was at the base of my spine, there were five discs that 'slipped'. I was totally rigid. I was either vertical or horizontal and the thought of sitting was a nightmare. Eventually I managed to sit but my back was just completely knotted and bent like a piece of steel and wouldn't move at all. When standing the thought of even attempting to touch my knees, let alone my toes, was just a massively painful experience and something totally beyond my capabilities. I had no flexibility whatsoever. If I tried to lean forward I just couldn't move. So I started to use any situation to encourage a little bit of flexibility to come back by creating a little physical tension, nothing significant and certainly not forcing it when I could. This could be when I was washing my hands at the sink. When I was waiting for a kettle to boil by holding the kitchen work surface. Sometimes I would lean against a door frame and use that as the support. At times it was like trying to bend a piece of steel, nothing was happening. But I kept trying and eventually a little bit of flexibility started to come back. I wouldn't say necessarily without pain at times but I was making the opportunity whenever I went to do something. Because a risk from a flexibility point of view is that you brace yourself so much that you don't bend or do anything because of your back pain and the rest of you starts to stiffen up as well.

Once I had started to get a little more resigned to my condition and less frightened I started to make sure that other parts of my body that were okay were kept flexible.

Hands, fingers, knuckle joints, arms, shoulders, elbows – all these needed to be kept in good working order so I developed a routine of making sure that I looked after these areas. Moving my neck where you can just bend your head a little. When sitting I could flex my feet, ankle, move my leg, stretch my knee. Maybe when you're sitting down just moving your leg a little bit to try and flex your knee. Keeping the rest of your body moving was hugely valuable and stopped those parts starting to stiffen up and lose tone. It also made me realise exactly where the problem I had was centred. Whilst not a pleasant finding it was valuable to know where I had to focus and also eased the stress in other parts of my body. I also found it eased the stress in my mind as I now knew that it was not everywhere in my body that was affected. I do add that none of these finding are massive in themselves but as I started to eliminate other concerns the overall stress level eased and I could focus on getting better rather than managing my stress.

A significant part of my stress came from not knowing what was wrong. I realised that I had a major problem but as the pain was across the whole of my back and I had pain right down to my feet, through my groin and knees – I really did not know what the real problem was. In principle I knew I had a back problem but I was unsure of the extent of the problem.

I had been to see a physiotherapist who refused to even touch me because of the state I was in. My general practitioner, who was excellent, referred me to a chiropractor. The chiropractor gave me a very clear message that he could do nothing, fully expecting I would never walk properly again. Eventually I came across a neurosurgeon who was a leader in his field of dealing with back problems without surgery. I know he's retired now but he told me that provided I did not do anything dramatically harsh to my back, I would not damage it anymore. He gave me the confidence to know I could get better. I was frightened about the amount of pain I was in and very stressed because of this pain. His reassurance that I needed to exercise and stretch stating that "it will hurt but it's not doing any more damage" really helped me reduce my anxiety.

I started to get my back a little bit more mobile by just testing it out in different places. When I was in a chair or when I was standing up, sometimes leaning against the wall or a work surface, slowly just by applying a little gentle pressure to get it moving it all helped. At times I will admit it hurt and almost encouraged me to go that little bit further without over doing it. Over time the flexing clearly started to create more movement in my back. Before it was so knotted and so tense I couldn't physically move it at all but slowly flexibility started to return.

I had done some yoga a few years before and I thought it could be a good idea to restart using one of the books I had bought. The problem was my yoga book was quite heavy to lift so I asked a friend to put it on a work surface so I could periodically just turn a page over and read different sections. By lying on the floor and doing certain yoga postures very, very gently started to help enormously. Linking the yoga with the meditation helped me relax and I found my stress levels also reduced. The yoga also helped my movement and flexibility to increase. At this time my pain level also increased but as I was becoming more mobile and my back flexibility had started to increase I seemed to be able to bear more pain as I knew I was developing a more normal lifestyle, and could see my return for the effort I was making. It made me feel more confident about the future and about what I was doing and, because of the reassurance from the neurosurgeon, I was not inflicting any more harm on myself.

I have seen many people with back problems who are so frightened of their problem that they do nothing. There is almost a resignation that now they have a back problem nothing can be done – it is chronic and that is the way life has to be. At worst this becomes a self-fulfilling prophecy because if the person sits and does nothing the muscles will start to deteriorate and waste away, posture starts to deteriorate, and the person starts to put on weight. Often to combat their stress they eat comforting food, which makes matters worse as they increase in bulk, which is more difficult and tiring to carry around.

I fought through this because I thought flexibility was important. I had never been a particularly flexible person and realised that this was part of my problem. I developed a regime in the morning and the evening to make sure that my non-back areas had a workout so they would be kept flexible and moving. Something as simple as clenching your fists and opening them out just to loosen up your hands will stop them getting stiff, and at worst arthritic before their time. It is worth creating your own regime and making sure you stick to it twice a day. All these small things help reduce the stress in your body.

Yoga

I did find it a little strange the first time I went to a yoga class because in the western world it tends to be ladies who do yoga and not men. Interestingly, in the eastern world it tends to be men not ladies. I was one man in a class of twenty ladies, I was as stiff as a board and in a lot of discomfort and pain and they were absolutely delightful. Some of the ladies could bend themselves double – amazing and in my condition quite humbling!

As mentioned in chapter 6 and 7 I value yoga and found the classes wonderful at de-stressing me and fantastic in helping my body become more flexible. Simply listening and watching the teacher explain the exercise position and then take up the position myself and applying a little extra stretch from what I could initially do caused no damage and increased strength and flexibility.

The key thing about flexibility exercises is they are not a once a week activity. I do my standard exercises twice a day. They don't take long and can easily be integrated in the normal routine of the day. Flexibility exercises can actually be done on the way to work, whilst showering, while you are waiting for the kettle to boil or the toast to pop up, on the way home from work, when you're doing your shopping, in the supermarket, while you're in the car and many other places too.

There are some exercises I have identified elsewhere in the book which take only a short time to do each day. Is it worth it? I think you don't have a choice and the length of time it takes is nothing compared with the discomfort and the debility you may have if you didn't do them. Certainly every time I stop doing my flexibility exercises and other daily exercises, and especially my flexibility exercises, I have paid the price. It is easy to integrate into each and every day.

ACTION

- If you feel stressed write down everything you are getting stressed about.

- What are you going to do to reduce any feeling of being stressed – breathing exercises, encouraging those who are close to enjoy things that they usually do, acknowledging the ability to work and speak with your employer?

- What are the small things you can start to do straight away to rebuild your confidence? There are many things you can do, what are they?
- If you are on medication what are you going to do to reduce and then eliminate this?

- Can you reduce stress through meditation?

- Consider your flexibility and relaxation – can you join a yoga class?

Chapter 11

Home and Work: Advice to speed recovery

Furniture

A bold statement I know but most furniture in the home is not conducive to high quality back care! So what do I mean? Generally chairs are the wrong shape. Three piece suites are often the wrong shape and frequently too soft. Beds are either too hard, too soft, too low and occasionally too high.

But the answer is not to go on a spending spree, which few people can afford, it is to learn how to use the furniture you currently have. It may require the odd additional item to help make life easier or to replace an item or two to ensure that you can treat your back well when at home. I do not advocate the mass change of things though as it will create a haven at home and a nightmare anywhere else. It is better to learn to live with the furniture that we encounter both at home and when elsewhere so we are able to live a life where we can manage with what there is.

I find it sad when I go to someone's home to find it full of special equipment and specialist furniture – how do they cope when they go out?!? Also their home may have lost some of that 'normal' look and homely feel as much of the equipment has an institutional look to it.

The sitting room

There are many nightmares of furniture that I have seen which are totally destined to create serious posture based problems. The three piece suite is the prime culprit as many are very soft when you sit in them. When you are fit you may feel comfortable but if you look at the posture of anyone sitting in this type of suite you will see that their knees are higher than their hips and they have a reclined posture. The strain of getting out of this type of seat is enormous even for fit people and whilst they may spring out of it, it does take a significant toll on their body to do this. Consider this for anyone suffering with back problems, the strain of getting out of this type of sitting position is huge – you may know this at your own personal cost due to the pain that you suffer when you get out of such a seat. It will also be very noticeable by the fact that you are stiff and it is difficult to move when you want too. Your posture is very poor when you attempt to stand up and quite probably the pain you experience has increased.

Some three piece suites are very good because they are higher, a little 'formal' but to many people they seem rather old fashioned. Leather suites are very fashionable and a significant problem is the fact that you slide on the seat. This means at times you are unable to sit for any length of time without wriggling and shuffling around to get yourself comfortable. The best type of scat to sit in, especially when you are in the early stage of back based problems, is one where the seat is quite formal. The back is high and supportive, there are arms on either side enabling you to rise from the seat using the added strength of your arms.

When visiting friends and family it is quite usual to be offered what they consider to be the "most comfortable and best seat" in the house. BE VERY CAREFUL! If it looks as if your knees will be higher than you hips when seated, and there is no access to at least one arm, say NO – this is the wrong type of seat to be sitting in. Do not feel obliged or think you may upset the person who is offering the best seat in the house. Ask for a higher chair that you are likely to find more comfortable. I have found that most people are a little concerned that the seat will be uncomfortable. I can assure you that having tried and failed to get comfortable and then suffered in many "best seats in the house" I will never ever accept a seat unless I know it is good for me. Eventually I found that people do not take offence. In fact I used to ask, ideally, for a carver dining chair (a dinning chair with arms), or if there was not

118

one available a dining chair. I would also ask for it to be placed next to something firm that I could hold and know it would help me to stand when I want to get up. Do not be swayed into sitting in a seat that it soft and unsupportive. I can assure you that sitting in the wrong type of seat will, at worst, increase your recovery time. You will never improve your back health by sitting in the wrong type of chair. (If someone does not have a good carver chair or dining chair then an alternative is a good garden patio chair.) If the seat is hard, a little too low or cold sit on, use a cushion or pillow.

Bedroom

A very soft bed is no good for quality back health. A very hard bed is not good for quality back health either. The best type of bed that you can get is supportive and reasonably firm. It should not compress significantly when you sit on the edge. It should also not be too low down.

I also found a duvet and fitted base sheet worked best. Traditional sheets seemed to get untucked too easily and sheets and a blanket always ended up tying me in knots.

It is useful in the early stages of recovery from a major back problem to have a dining chair preferably a carver, near the bed. This is because when you have eventually got out of bed, especially if you suffer a lot of pain in doing this, it is an excellent "half way house" and a good place just to settle before you go to the bathroom or get dressed.

At one point water beds became very fashionable. They are a nightmare to get onto and off if you suffer with serious back problems!

Kitchen

If you are fortunate to have a large kitchen where you have a dining table and chair – great. Use it. If your kitchen is somewhat smaller it is useful to have a bar stool or similar so you can perch on it for temporary recovery whilst you are preparing food or a drink. If you live by yourself, when you are struggling to move around your home this may be the only place where you can eat or drink. The risk of taking hot food, and especially hot drinks around the house should be avoided. You have enough problems already so whilst it is not very dignified to perch or sit in the kitchen to drink or eat it is fine. And far better than having your dinner end up on the floor or a scalding hot drink poured down your front.

In the early stages of recovery it is an excellent way of making sure that you do eat properly as mentioned in the food section of this book. Sometimes it is better to accept your short term limitations so that you can start to do the normal things of life and from those successes move forward. I do stress not to adapt your home unless absolutely necessary. My goal for you is to live a life where you don't need special equipment at all.

Study/work station

You may work from home or your work requires that you have access to a computer at home. You may even get a lot of pleasure from writing, reading or using a computer. This is a risky area for good quality back care. To have the wrong type of chair can be very damaging to your back. To have the wrong height of desk can also be very damaging to your back. The ideal chair to sit at your desk is where your knees are slightly lower than your hips. It will, preferably have arms to support your forearms whilst working at the desk. In an idea world it will also have a very supportive back and head restraint.

The perfect type of office chair is not cheap, but if you intend to spend significant parts of your day at your desk it is a very sound investment to consider. Do ensure it has wheels, and additionally a variety of adjustments that can be made to suit you so you get a perfect seating position. It is wise to invest in appropriate equipment for key areas. You may find that it can be wheeled elsewhere in the house to provide high quality seating during the initial stages of your recovery. Also note that to move the chair around it is better to have a hard surface or place a special thick plastic mat under the chair wheels to both aid movement and also avoid damage to a carpet.

Desk

This should be at a height that is neither too high nor too low. Desks can be increased in height by putting something under each of the legs. I have been told that the reason most desks are the same height is because originally they were made to go through a standard door frame! Clearly we are all of different heights so this is a case where one size should not suit all.

If you measure a desk or table you will find that the height is 29 inches (approx 73 centimetres). The desk I use for my computer is 31.5 inches high (80 centimetres) almost 10% higher. So I suggest you have a good look at your desk – is it the right height for you? Do you have a chair that is also the right height?

If you spend much time at a desk this is an absolutely crucial area to review. Any changes you make to correctly fit your needs and own height will be well rewarded. If there are other people who also use the same desk you will need a chair that can increase or decrease in height. You may also find that a foot rest accommodates shorter members of the household or office.

Working at a desk

To safeguard your back and to aid its recovery it is always wise to have all the critical items that you use within easy reach. A simple example of something that is wrong would be a telephone or pen holder that it just a little too far out of reach so that you have to stretch every time you answer the phone or get a pencil. This is bad news because it will inevitably induce an unnecessary twist into your back every time you reach. For many people these small irritations have been the start of a back problem.

This is not a section about total health but clearly be minded of the need for good quality light and ventilation too.

As an additional point do bear in mind that we can get easily absorbed when using computers or engrossed in work or reading for prolonged periods of time. Our posture takes a poor second place as our mind is elsewhere. There are some key points here:

- Firstly, do make sure that you maintain a healthy intake of water.
- Secondly, break for meal times.
- Thirdly, perhaps most importantly, do stand and move around on a regular basis to avoid getting set in one position and encourage your back to keep moving.
- Fourthly, use a timer to remind yourself to move – see below.

In the initial stages I would recommend that you stand and move, even if it is only across the room and back, every twenty minutes. I have found a useful trick to deploy at home is to get a noisy egg timer and place it out of reach and set it for twenty minutes, that way you will have to get up, to shut it up! Also when you are there stopping it, you can reset it for the next twenty minutes.

I am aware of people who have significant back based problems which they have had for many years. Frequently this is because they sit for prolonged periods of time without getting up, often using a poorly sized desk and inappropriate chair. Once they start to move on a more regular basis their speed of recovery increases. If they also make sure they have the desk and chair of the correct height they can improve their recovery still further. It can be difficult for them, it may be painful, they will ache but the decision is theirs to start on a road to a better quality of life. Is now a good time to review your desk, chair and working conditions? If you are taking your recovery seriously you know the answer!

Now you have read this you owe it to those in your household who don't have a bad back at the moment to ensure that you are doing what you can to help them too.

Bathroom

Firstly, be very careful of wet slippery floors as a sudden slip could cause a setback to your recovery. When going somewhere new do get used to checking the flooring and the likelihood that it could be slippery. Ceramic tiles, wooded floors, especially laminate and vinyl, are all surfaces that should be treated with caution and respect.

If you see a loose mat on the floor this could make things even more hazardous. Tread with extreme care, or move it!

Bath v shower

It is important to maintain high quality personal hygiene and the thought of a long soak in a hot bath to relax painful back muscles is wonderful. In the early stages of back problems a bath may well be a step too far and just not possible, in which case a shower may be the only option. Do not risk a bath if you have some concerns as you may get stuck, especially if you enjoy a long soak. Do bear in mind too that if you have a bath the soap will make the surface more slippery so be extremely careful when you get out. With a bad back we tend to be more clumsy anyway and less able to counter any slip.

Two important points with a bath:

- Make sure you get out whilst the water is still quite warm as you will stiffen up if it starts to cool too much.
- Get out with water still in the bath – it will make your weight feel less. Getting out of an empty bath requires much more strength.

Some showers have doors which open inwards – there is an inherent <u>danger</u> in these if you have a major back problem and collapse against the door, as it will be very difficult for anyone else to get in and help you. So be very careful if your shower is of this design. If the door opens outwards there is less risk of you getting stuck. If you really have a significant problem and mobility is very poor, whilst unsightly it may well be worthwhile having a hand grip installed so that you can support yourself in a vertical position and can shower. Also note that when soaped up a shower does become slippery so do take care at this time and if necessary fit a rubber suction mat to stand on – just ensure it does not block the plug hole otherwise you may run the risk of a small flood!

When you step out of the shower be careful not to slip, especially if your floor is of a hard surface. Mats to stand on can be a real nightmare and do make sure that any that are on the floor won't slip. Think of a lovely dry towel on a dry shiny surface – a major hazard, so don't even consider it!

If your shower is over the bath it is critical, unless you have a non slip surface, to use a rubber suction mat to stand on (again avoiding covering the plug hole). Also consider fitting a hand grip if you have nothing to hold on to securely.

When you are in the shower make sure you clean yourself fully and also take the opportunity to massage your back and any other aching muscles while you are there. It is much easier when you are wet. Also do your stretches.

Wash hand basin

When we are in the early stages of back problem we will cling onto anything that is remotely secure just to support ourselves. Do make sure that your wash hand basin will take the strain as you can imagine the risk of it becoming loose and falling on your feet! Some are surprisingly loose too so, especially if you are somewhere unfamiliar, don't assume the wash hand basin is really secure.

I will guarantee that there is no wash hand basin that feels at the right height. Therefore to wash, shave (obviously for men) and clean your teeth it may be a messy business! So put a hand towel around your neck while you do these things. Adopt a semi crouching stance will help you get closer to the basin – a little like the way an ape or monkey would stand! Reminder – don't forget to stretch whilst doing these daily ablutions!

Toilet

Where possible try not to adapt your toilet by using a seat riser attachment unless you are very tall. I am always keen to retain a 'normal' appearance in your home. I do suggest that you ensure that the lid is a firm one so that the toilet can be used as a seat. The effort of using the toilet at a normal height will be a beneficial part of your longer term recovery and also, and this is a key point, it will get you used to using a standard toilet wherever you go. If you adapt your own home toilet it means that every other toilet will be a challenge – this way it conditions you to using toilets wherever you happen to be.

If you **really** must use a seat riser attachment so that you can cope in the early stages of your problem set a date when you will remove it. Diarise the date too so you remember to remove it – if you don't remove it you cheat yourself and the people around you as you are delaying your recovery.

Two important tips:

- Tip one – you may find in your own bathroom that there is solid support to lower and raise yourself from the toilet. This is guaranteed not always to be the case elsewhere. If you are suffering seriously with your mobility take one and preferably two solid walking sticks with you.

- Tip two – put adequate toilet paper in your pocket before you sit on the loo. If you have not got a suitable pocket (a perfect pocket is a breast pocket on a shirt), tuck the toilet paper where you will be able to reach it when you are seated. Again it is guaranteed that the position of the toilet paper holder will, in many cases, mean it is out of reach or you have to twist to access it, all of which can be massively painful and at such times as this you are trying to maintain a little dignity and a high level of personal hygiene.

  - Another way is to take a box of tissues with you.
  - I found that the small packets of tissues (10 in a pack), which you can get almost everywhere, were very useful to carry in a pocket. (Often one is rather clumsier than usual and they are useful for many eventualities no matter where you are – they make good standby serviettes too.)

NOTE: Do not skip good hygiene standards when you are in the bathroom as an upset stomach is the last thing you want at these challenging times. Make sure you also wash hands with plenty of soap and water.

It is now possible to get a hand gel that kills germs and whilst no replacement for good old fashioned washing it is a great standby for many situations. If you use a stick to get around when in the bathroom make sure the handle is kept hygienic too.

Furniture – Office

Many of the points mentioned regarding home/study/work station applies in the office. There is one significant difference and that is at work you will probably be seated for significantly longer periods of time over the day, especially if you have an office based job. The importance of a good work place assessment on your return to work after being diagnosed with major back problems if very important.

This work place assessment should cover seating, desk height and position, any computer equipment and associated equipment, filing and services that you will be using. I would suggest that whilst aiming to make your work place as suitable for you as possible, ensure it is not created into some massively specialised area of the office. Unless, of course, your complaint and condition means that the probability of you returning to normal fitness is unlikely. It may be that in the short term after a very major problem you will require specialist facilities. I do encourage you to remove these as soon as you possibly can so that you get used to living in the world everyone lives in. Don't end up working somewhere that does not allow you to start to condition yourself to working with the compromises that are inherent in other work areas. Areas that we will visit either within our own organisation or anywhere else.

I do stress that a key part of getting better is to be mobile. When at work do not sit for hours on end. Get up and walk a few feet and then sit down again, stretch, 'wriggle' in your seat. I will not be prescriptive although a suggestion is to stand up every 20 minutes. Have a little walk every 40 minutes, have a longer walk at 90 minutes and add some stretches into this routine. How do you remember to do this – simply get yourself a small kitchen timer as I mentioned before. This time one that is not too noisy or use the vibrate mode on your mobile phone and put it in your pocket or close by on your desk. Colleagues nearby will soon get annoyed with the loud regular interruptions, so be respectful – but do use something. Don't feel embarrassed by this, likewise don't make a show and become the martyr moaning about the pain you are in and being a pain in the neck to colleagues!

Cloakroom facilities

Take a similar approach to those that you would at home. The one area that can be a challenge is drying hands using a wall mounted dryer. The sheer pain of standing still long enough to dry your hands can be an excuse not to wash your hands. Do not ever forego high quality hygiene. Consider taking paper towels with you to work for this eventuality. Or accepting that using a hand dryer gives you the opportunity to improve posture and do exercises that will aid your recovery.

Doors

At home it can be a good idea to leave inside doors open unless it creates too much of a draft. If they are fire doors though you may have to reconsider this statement. Don't lock bathroom doors from the inside unless you have to just in case you need some unexpected assistance.

Sometimes office doors, which are almost always spring loaded, are very heavy. You are aiming to become self sufficient so do not always wait or expect others to open them for you. Develop your way of getting through these without hurting yourself or inconveniencing others. A way is to gently lean on the door and slowly walk it open. Be careful that the door springing back does not destabilise you or hurt others.

Revolving doors – BE CAREFUL. The main concern is someone else "driving" at a speed that is far too fast for you. If there is a side door next to the revolving door that is useable then use that. If you have no alternative and are in the early stages of recovery ask someone to help you. I had a very nasty experience when someone tried to go through at speed. Learn from my pain!

Floors

Many offices, especially those of large prestigious organisations, have wonderful polished floors. Tread carefully, especially if wet – they can be lethal. If you are used to wearing leather bottomed shoes reconsider this until you are surefooted again and think about wearing rubber bottomed shoes. Rubber soles are also prone to slip on wet shiny floors too, so take care. Clearly high heeled shoes are completely inappropriate and hopefully not even being considered.

Briefcase and carrying things

In the early stages of a major back pain episode you will not even think about carrying anything. As things start to improve this will be something to reintroduce. A few points – make sure any case and bag has been cleared of ALL junk and unnecessary items. If you are asking someone else to carry a bag for you don't make them carry more than is essential. You will also start to develop a good habit for the future. It is amazing just how much people do carry, much of which is not needed. A ladies handbag can be a very small with essentials only. A larger bag will encourage more to be carried so be warned!

Rather than use a lovely heavy leather case perhaps find a much lighter bag. Consider one that has a handgrip **and** a shoulder strap. Whilst not very professional for some office workers, a small rucksack can be good as it will help with posture if both straps are used. Don't overfill!

Lifts, stairs, escalator and moving floors

The automatic choice is to go for the lift as 'I have a back problem'. Don't – weight up the options first!

- Firstly consider the lift:

  My first choice when I needed to go up or down a large building, station or airport would usually be a lift/elevator. I would be very careful when I got in it to avoid anybody knocking me with trolleys or luggage. I would also tend to shy away into the corner of a lift, put my back to the side and try and make sure people didn't get too close. If you explain to people, they are generally very understanding.

  It never ceases to amaze me that when families and friends are travelling together there is an overwhelming enthusiasm to get everyone and everything in the lift at the same time. If you see such a crowd forming it may be wise to wait for the next lift.

- o Advantages include:
  - Can be quicker.
  - Saves you having to manage the stairs and the effort that will take.
  - Usually takes you to the main reception areas on each floor.
- o Disadvantages include:
  - It may be very busy and you will get knocked about when you get in/out.
  - If it is crowded then it may be awkward when you are in it.
  - The risk the doors could pose if they shut on you.
  - Getting trapped if it stops and the pain of having to stand for much longer than you bargained for.
  - If the lift is jerky this is a potential pain area.
  - If the lift does not align with the floor when it stops.
  - Being caught by peoples shopping or bags.

- Secondly consider the stairs:

  The stairs can be a very slow and painful journey but sometimes it is the only option. Sometimes it can be a great way to get some more exercise and practice and worth taking.

Do be aware of your security though as some stair wells are poorly lit, unclean and also attract people who are focussed on crime.

- o Advantages include:
  - You are in control.
  - You can stop.

- They are probably quieter.
- There is little probability of you getting trapped.
- It a great form of exercise.
  o Disadvantages include:
    - Usually slower.
    - The door to get into the stair wells may be on strong springs.
    - Are they used? – For both personal security reasons and also if you have a problem will someone find you?
    - They are often out of the main areas.

- Thirdly consider the escalators:

Escalators are an amazing invention for saving effort. When you have a bad back there is a major risk at the point of getting on and off one. It can be especially awkward if there are many people bustling around too.

At times I found I had to be downright rude to people and say 'can you give me space, I've got a bad back and need to get on here'. People become so absorbed in what they are doing that no one else seems to matter in their lives. They are in a rush. Sometimes late and little else seems to matter to them. Sometimes you can be very polite and it gets the result you want too – it all depends on when and where you are. If you are in any very busy city anywhere in the world people are living fast lives – especially at the rush hour. Many underground train systems the world over are accessed by escalators so my suggestion is avoid them at rush hour if you have a bad back and it is very painful.

In the early stages of my back pain problems I would not use escalators. Getting on and getting off was so painful.

  o Advantages include:
    - Saves effort.

- You can see what is going on around you.
- There is a handrail to hold.
- Easier than the stairs.
- Usually in a good location in a shop or shopping mall.
- Often rise from the reception of large offices.
  - o Disadvantages include:
    - Can be jerky.
    - Not always easy to get on and off.
    - If busy people can push you.
    - If you are standing on one side people rushing past can knock you or their bags hit you.

- Fourthly consider moving floors (these are often found at airports):

  They can be very good for moving through a building where there are large distances to cover. Once on them it is possible to walk on them too. They are usually in main thoroughfares so open and you can see what is going on around you. They are also good when you have luggage as it can just stand on the floor and if it has wheels provided they are in the line of travel are less difficult to get off when compared with an escalator – but there will always be a challenge at the end!

  - o Advantages include:
    - Can travel long distances with little effort.
    - They don't go too fast.
    - They tend to be smooth.
  - o Disadvantages include:
    - Getting on or off the floor.
    - Passengers late for their flight who run down them with bags flying around (Tip: stand in front of someone else and also

> stand sideways so you take up less room and keep your eyes and ears open.)
> - Slippery if wet.
> - Makes you lazy!

Obviously if it is a 50 storey building you are going up, there may be an easy decision to be made after all!!

ACTION

- Undertake an 'audit' of the furniture you use and establish what is good for your posture and what is not so good.

- Decide to only use the right furniture that will help you recover – and if necessary ask people to move things around so it works for you (and doesn't inconvenience everyone else!).

- Review your bathroom and shower – are there any hazards that need to be dealt with?

- Look at any adaptations around your home that you should consider removing as they are slowing your recovery.

- Make sure that you use opportunities to stretch when undertaking daily tasks such as cleaning teeth.

- Keep mobile and don't sit for periods longer than 40 minutes, and ideally 20 minutes.

- Clear out any bags you carry so they weigh as little as possible.

- Are you always using a lift or escalator when out – consider using the stairs to develop strength.

Chapter 11 - Home and Work: Advice to speed recovery

Chapter 12

Tested approaches to ease the hassle of travel

One of the biggest challenges when one has a problem back is simply getting around. Life, particularly after a major back problem can be dramatically different compared with how it was before. Even the simplest of journeys becomes a real challenge. I have identified below some of the methods that can be used to combat problems when travelling.

Walking

Walking is a key aspect of any normal daily life. Obviously the simple task of walking to a bathroom needs to be undertaken but for sufferers of a major back problem even this simple challenge is an enormous task. Sometimes, people will take every opportunity to avoid walking as it hurts. I would discourage this attitude and use the need for every errand to be part of your journey to recovery.

In the early stages of recovery it may be necessary to use a walking stick. I would suggest if you need to use a stick you do use two. This will ensure that your body is working in a balanced way and force it to start on the journey of recovery. If you are confined to a chair aim to get up at regular intervals and go for a short walk. This walk may only be across the room and back but do make the effort. I have seen many people who say they cannot move from the chair but spend the night in bed. If they can get to the chair and out of it this is a great start. They just need to do it more often! I found it horrifically painful to get out of a chair but knew that I had to for the basic functions of life. The realisation that I had the ability to get out of a chair, even if pain ridden, gave me the motivation to keep trying ways to make it less painful. In time I found ways and it became less painful.

I would stress it may not be comfortable but it is crucial to your recovery that you start to walk. No matter how hard, make the effort and don't avoid walking because it is painful. It is part of the recovery process.

Once the initial major problems are subsiding start to extend your walking on a regular basis, and where possible, without using a stick. If the ground is uneven consider taking two but clearly you will need to tread carefully.

Car – As a passenger

When I first had my major problem I didn't travel by car at all, it was not an option. When I did start my first stage was as a passenger in a car, when I could get in it. It is a challenge with some cars as the roof is low and there is not enough flexibility in one's back to bend. I found it amazing just how much I learnt about car design and often, it seems, design is more important than function.

In the early stages it may be excruciatingly painful to get into a car. Inevitable for many of us, the use of a car is a way of life and the main means by which we can get around. It may be that getting to a doctor's appointment will require a car journey. The first challenge is actually getting into a car and the way to do this is as follows:

1. Ensure the car is parked on as flat a surface as possible and the door can be opened as wide as possible.
2. Place a clean polythene bag on the seat edge to sit on.
3. Aim to sit sideways on the car seat with your legs outside, back inside and sitting on the polythene bag.
4. When lowering yourself into the car, because your back is rigid, be extremely careful not to hit your head on the upper edges of the door opening by the roof. Once you

have sat on the edge of the seat aim to slide on the polythene bag onto the seat.

5. Now slowly grab anything you can to support yourself and in a twisting motion, on the polythene bag, aim to move your feet into the foot well of the car so you are facing forward and not twisted.

6. Adjust the car seat as much as you can to get as comfortable as possible. Do make sure that the back rest is in a reasonably vertical position and not reclining significantly. This is because of both safety and support for you on the journey.

7. Fasten seatbelt and ensure it is reasonably tight around you.

8. When the car door is closed brace yourself as much as possible so that the bumps and bends on the car journey are as painless as possible.

9. Ask the driver to be considerate of your situation whilst not causing a road hazard to others. The key pain areas are potholes, rapid and sudden acceleration, poor gear changes, jerky braking and fast cornering. If possible ask the driver to give you advanced warning of any action they are going to take.

Car – As a driver

First and foremost do ensure that you are safe to drive as you may well be uninsured if you drive whilst unwell or on certain medication. Many a drunk driver believes that they can drive well so don't fool yourself about your ability.

To get into the car use the same procedure as if you are a passenger – but remove the plastic bag once you are seated as it will be slippery and could cause you loss of control in an emergency.

Now check the following before you even start the engine:

- Can you press the brake pedal hard for an emergency stop?
- Are you struggling to depress the clutch for a gear change in a manual car, or is it easy enough?
- Can you reach all of the controls easily?
- Can you twist sufficiently to see around you properly, say, at a blind junction?

If you are uncertain you are not safe to drive – so don't! You are endangering yourself and others.

Also ask yourself the acid test question – 'as a passenger would I like this person to drive me and would I feel safe?' If the answer is 'no' don't drive!

In the early stages of back problems, if you drive, under all circumstances ensure that you stop after approximately thirty minutes. Get out of the car to have a short walk and a stretch before getting back into the car and continuing with your journey. This may seem excessive but it is always recommended that no one drives for more than two hours when they are fit and alert. **You are not fit and your level of alertness will fade quickly if you have back pain.**

It is also important to change your position so that you can start to develop a healthier body. Sitting in one fixed position, as we tend to in a car, is not conducive to a speedy recovery. Do take note of this point as it is valuable in ensuring you are both safe on the road and you do not over stress your body because of the journey.

You may not realise it but the movement of the car creates significant motion around the spine and on the core muscles. This will cause you to ache, and is one of the reasons why we ache when travelling. If the car suspension is very firm this will exacerbate the problem and you may find a stop after less than thirty minutes is more comfortable.

Racing cars have very firm suspension. Racing drivers are usually very fit and strong because they have to be to endure the demands racing a car places on them. To a lesser extent the same is true of a normal road car.

Public transport

Train

Travelling on a train when experiencing a bad back is a major problem and in the early stages of recovery should probably be avoided.

Initially, you have to get to the rail station and that will be by car, walking or by bus. Once at the station getting around may prove to be a problem and do take care if it is a busy time of day as other fellow passengers will be in a rush and you are likely to be knocked.

Many trains have automatic doors. Where the door is non automatic be very careful, as the weight of the doors is considerable. In the past you may have just grabbed the handle, twisted it and then pulled the door open. With a back problem this is not easy and the sheer pain will be horrible. So be careful.

See whether someone else is going to open it. Whilst I advocate you become independent there are certain times when it is better to ask or let other people do things for you. At times it is not possible for others to help so when you get to the door acknowledge that it will probably be dirty, are you wearing gloves? Once you have twisted the handle, put your other hand on the carriage and pull open the door carefully.

Do this for two reasons – one is it provides a uniform pressure across the top part of your back which will potentially reduce the pain that you'll incur when you open the door. And the second one is if it opens quickly, or it won't open, you can balance the pressure and avoid any suddenness. Make sure you open it wide enough and use both hands. Also use both hands to get on the train and go one step at a time into the carriage.

If you are carrying anything, and I'm referring to something even quite small, leave it on the platform whilst opening the door, then pick the bag up and put it inside the train, then with completely empty hands get in the train. This applies to all trains whether automatic doors or manual doors. It is best, if you have got to have a bag, to use a shoulder bag so you can just slip it over your shoulder so both hands are free.

If you think the train is going to move before you've got to your seat be hugely careful. Use whatever support you need to help yourself down the carriage because I will guarantee if that train starts while you are walking to your seat it will hurt. Be prepared to brace yourself, from the jolt of the train, when it starts to move.

Be careful where you sit and if possible make sure you have adequate leg space. There are pros and cons between the inside seat and the aisle seat. Inside seats are good because you don't get knocked by fellow passengers moving down the aisle. However if you are on a train for any length of time and want to stretch you may not be able to easily get out. If it is a commuter train and always very busy my suggestion is sit away from the aisle. If you are on a long distance train journey sit by the aisle so you can get up every 20 minutes or so, have a gentle walk and a gentle stretch around. Even if only one or two seats down the aisle, and back, to keep your body moving. Once a train is in motion it is possible to carefully get up from your seat – do take note of when you are expecting the train to slow, especially for a station.

When in a train I would suggest you travel with your back to the engine so if it does brake quickly you are not going to shoot forward. Also if you have your back to the engine you are in a much better position if there are more jerks, particularly if it's stopping. I tended to brace myself against the seat arms. When in the seat wedge yourself in so you can brace yourself with your elbows. Occasionally the passenger next to you may want the arm rest too, but quite often a polite conversation with the person to explain your problem can be very helpful.

A tip – I found that, if it was a longer journey, by bracing my elbows into the arms of the seat I could ease myself up out of the seat – not necessarily by very much – but enough to take the pressure onto my elbows. By doing so it took the pressure from my lower back and created a little stretch in my spine. A little easing of the pressure and it felt like a light massage.

Crucially, keep flexible by moving. Don't wedge yourself in and get stuck for hours on end in the same position even if you are comfortable. Acknowledge the fact that keeping flexible is important. If it's an old rattley train that bounces around you probably won't be doing anything else other than coping with the journey. If it's a much smoother more modern train it is a good idea to take something to distract yourself. A good book or a hobby that you have. An iPod would be fine, but don't get too absorbed so that you sit for too long without moving. If you don't move you will pay the price when you have to start to move again.

Bus

The most difficult parts are getting on and off the bus.

Most bus drivers sit near the door where you get on. With those that don't there is usually a conductor who will supervise people getting on and off. I have found almost without exception, if you are pleasant to the driver or conductor before you get on and explain that you have a back problem, they will wait till you are seated before they drive off.

Look into the bus and see or ask if there are any seats. If you have a really bad back it is not a good idea to stand on a bus journey. There are lots of stops and starts and it can be very jerky too. You will know yourself if it is wiser to wait for the next one where there may be a seat.

Aim to sit close to the door with a seat in front of you and also near a bell push, so you can press it yourself to alert the driver that you want to get off. I would suggest avoiding seats that face sideways. If you are not near the bell push, make sure you are close to someone who can do it for you by asking them. The last thing you want is to wander down the central aisle ready for your bus stop whilst the bus is in motion.

If your journey is short and the bus is not busy, I suggest sitting on the outside seat next to the aisle. If the bus is busy and it's a slightly longer journey, sit on the inside near the window.

If the bus has two decks sit down stairs. Firstly it saves the need to use the stairs. Secondly the bus sways more upstairs than downstairs. This may seem only a small difference but I can assure you from experience the difference is noticeable!

If you have a season ticket I suggest you put it in a pocket you can get at easily, or in an easily accessible part of a handbag so you avoid dithering around when you get on the bus. It could mean the difference between you sitting down before the bus moves off. If you're using cash make sure that you have the right change, if possible, so that you pay quickly and sit down.

Keep luggage to a minimum and if possible don't have any. A shoulder bag is easier providing it is not heavy.

There are normally lots of poles and bars on a bus to steady yourself, so use them. Use the edge of the seat backs too.

When you sit down, wedge yourself so the motion of the bus can be made less uncomfortable. I found I had to sit differently on a bus when compared with a train. You need to brace yourself to take account of the acceleration away from bus stops and traffic lights, the braking for stops and traffic lights and also the general ebb and flow the bus will encounter in traffic. On a train there is no traffic so once it is in motion the next time it slows is when it is nearing the next station. A very different experience from road travel.

The way I braced myself was to hold the top of the seat in front with one hand and the side with the other. Many people thought it was odd but I found it the most effective way of easing the painful parts of the irregular driving speeds when on a bus. It made the ebb and the flow of the journey far less painful.

A useful tip is to be alert to what is going on around you. If you can see a traffic light is changing from green to red you know the bus will have to slow and stop so anticipate what you need to do to be comfortable. Likewise, when you see the traffic lights change from red to green, anticipate again what is the most comfortable action for you. If you can see the road in front of the bus you can keep an eye out for what is happening and know what action the bus driver will make. This is one of the reasons why it is useful to sit near the front of the bus.

Air travel

Certainly in the initial stage of a major back problem, flying is probably out of the question unless needed for emergency reasons. It was not something I would consider and my recommendation if you have a major back problem is don't fly.

When I started to get a little better I thought it was something I could do and when you live in the UK, as lovely as it is, it is not renowned for great weather. To enjoy a vacation somewhere the sun is likely to be guaranteed has attraction.

I would stress even to this day I am very mindful of aircraft travel and the impact it may have on my back. This is not because I have a problem anymore as my problems are pretty much cured because I have taken responsibility and dealt with it. I have flown around the world by plane. I have been on very long, long haul flights – the longest flight I've ever been on was a 14 hour non-stop from London in England to Tokyo in Japan and I had no problems. So flying is an option and there are ways to look after your back during such flights.

Once you start to regain some mobility and are able to travel by car, bus or train you may wish to fly again. This could be for business or pleasure and there are many things that you can do to make things much easier for you.

I get very annoyed when people abuse systems that are put in place for people with special needs. One of the services that I have found to be valuable, albeit of variable standards the world over, is the airport buggy service. If you have a genuine problem they can be brilliant for taking the strain and stress out of airports. Some airports are vast and the distances you have to travel from check in to the departure gate can be large. Or when you land the terminal exit is so far away it could ruin your trip. If you do have a problem the people who operate the service are usually delighted to be able help whenever they possibly can. You can short-circuit the queues as the thought of standing up for 20 minutes, half an hour, an hour to go through customs and security can be hideously painful and just totally impossible for somebody with a really bad back problem.

Some tips:

- Pack lightly – really consider what you need to take. I can travel for a month with barely any more than I take for a long weekend away and look very smart all of the time. The amount of luggage some people take is quite ridiculous and during major security alerts it focuses the mind on what you really need!

- Travel in very comfortable clothes – and this is not an opportunity to be scruffy! Comfortable clothes, which may have a slightly elasticised waistband, are crease resistant and easy to mix layers to keep you at the right temperature. Ideally a little loose fitting so you can feel more comfortable. Have shoes that will slide off easily and importantly slide back on easily too. So avoid lace up shoes – feet swell on long flights and also having to bend to lace them up in a confined space with a bad back could be painful. (There is a mixed view on this issue though and some medical people advise keeping shoes on and laced up to help avoid vascular problems.) Be sensible about what you're wearing so you are genuinely very comfortable and presentable.

- Pack any medication or essential travel items in your hand luggage. I would also suggest a set of underwear just in case your luggage gets lost so you can manage another day without worrying too much.

When you are on a plane the physiology of your body changes. Your body swells due to the pressure changes in the cabin, your feet can puff up so shoes feel less comfortable. It is an interesting experiment to see how much an empty plastic water bottle with the cap screwed on changes shape during a flight – if it does that to a bottle think what happens to your body! That is one of the reasons I would reconsider flying when you are in the early stages of recovering from a bad back.

You need to drink a lot of water when you're on an aeroplane, with the consequence that you need to go to the toilet more often. So, understand that you need to be capable of being mobile on an aeroplane and if you find the trips to the toilet are difficult at home it will be worse on a plane. The recommendation when flying is to sit and wear your seat belt – just sitting all the time will cause you to stiffen up and be even less mobile. During turbulence you are not allowed to get up from your seat so if you are confined to sitting for long periods you may really suffer. Consider this before flying and don't let the enthusiasm for the vacation or importance of the business meeting take precedence.

We all have heard of the horror stories where people have been stranded for hours. Make sure you are prepared for delays and capable of coping with them, just in case.

When on the plane, and in the airport beforehand, if you have been there some while make sure that you do some exercises. With the greater awareness of DVT (deep vein thrombosis), we know we should be exercising. But how many of us do?! Look around on a flight and you will see few people undertaking any exercises.

Long before awareness of exercising while airborne was raised you would see me doing a whole range of exercises – moving my feet, my arms, my hands, looking an absolute idiot at times by stretching to keep myself flexible. Trying to put my head between my knees, and generally having a good stretch. Even if seated there is a lot you can do and the fact that you are wearing comfortable and not too tight clothing means you can exercise and stretch easily. If you are on a business trip it is better to dress less formally on the flight and change at the airport into more formal wear when you get to your destination.

When on the plane if possible get up frequently and walk about.

If you are on a large plane, especially if it is a long-haul flight, the cabin staff are generally a little bit more lenient about you walking around. Use the opportunity to go for a walk, to get a glass of water, or for a stretch.

Within the privacy of the toilet you can do some quite unusual stretches, which you probably wouldn't wish to do in the public area of the aeroplane – so moving around is pretty important.

Seat choice can be important too. If you have a back problem you will not or should not be allowed to sit by the emergency exit even though they have more space. People in these seats should be able bodied so they can be useful in an emergency. So don't lie about your condition on the pretext of getting more space. It is better to explain when checking in that you have a problem and the staff will be as helpful as possible. It may be that you need to sit closer to the toilet, or prefer an aisle seat or window seat. Ask.

Alternatively find out what type of plane you are travelling in and see whether you can check the floor plan/seating plan on the internet before you go. Or when you get to the checking in point, do highlight the problem you have and ask if there is any seat with a little more leg room, where you can sit safely without inconveniencing other people. Getting to the check-in a little earlier can be useful, or if possible advance booking your seats.

Do bear in mind that the bulkhead curves, so if you are in the window seat of a small plane you will have less leg room than the middle or the outer seat. So choose wisely, if you are a small person that probably doesn't matter – if you are a tall person that may be important to you. Remember, if it is a long flight and you have a really problematic back you will need to go to the toilet and it will be more difficult to get out of your seat. In this case it is far better to be in the aisle seat – but do acknowledge that you are going to have the trolleys and other people walking past. Plus anybody on the inside seat will ask you to move as they need the toilet.

On an overnight flight I have fallen asleep only to be woken when someone is politely trying to avoid waking me by climbing over me on their way to the toilet. If they had fallen the pain with my back would have been awful.

So where do you sit? My suggestions are:

- On a short hop flight – next to the window.
- On a midsized plane on a medium length day flight – next to the aisle.
- On a long haul flight – if there are three sets of seats with a central bank, choose the outer seat of the central bank so anyone who needs to get out can go the opposite direction from you.

All aircraft seats have arms so use them to ease yourself up periodically and stretch yourself. Use any pillow or cushions to make yourself as comfortable and as well supported as possible. All aircraft have spare cushions so ask the steward or stewardess for an extra one.

Now a word of warning – don't get so comfortable that you don't move for hours on end. I foolishly didn't move on one long-haul flight and realised after 3 hours I could not move without extreme pain. It took me quite a while and much discomfort to start to mobilise again. It is so easy to get involved in some music or a good book and let the time pass – set a timer if you need to and make sure you do some exercises regularly and get up for a walk even if only to the toilet. Use my pain for your gain!

Luggage

If you are travelling and need luggage, particularly if you're travelling with a companion, travel reasonably light between the two of you.

Swallow your pride and ask the other person to carry the bags. I was going on holiday with my wife in the 1980s and I got a lot of abuse because she carried the luggage and I didn't. I had to accept the situation. She was very supportive. Some people criticised me for not carrying the cases – I was recovering from having been in plaster for months and could not manage any weight. So, travel light, it eases the burden. Many suitcases have wheels, which certainly do make it a lot easier, although this is no reason to take more than you need.

When you drag a case or bag on wheels along you may well twist your body, so take care. Check to see if the handle or loop to pull the luggage is long enough – some cases only have short pulls so make it longer otherwise you will stoop and twist to pull it along which will cause wear and tear on your back.

At some point you will always have to lift luggage by hand even if it has wheel. Perhaps up stairs, when getting on or off transport, at the check-in at the airport, at your destination. Reclaiming luggage off the carousel can be an especially difficult event as it is moving and you need to pull cases off sideways. Often it is much wiser to use two lighter bags so they are evenly spread on both sides when you carry them, rather than one larger bag. Try things out before you finally pack for the journey and see what works best for you. And ask other people to help – most people are more than willing. If you have packed a hugely heavy bag I don't think it is fair on your fellow passengers to ask. So be minded of what you are asking other people to do on your behalf and also what your luggage says about you. If it is heavy, have you a real problem? If it is light your fellow passengers will probably be more understanding. Be congruent!

A point on security – be a little bit careful when you are in foreign countries, or somewhere unfamiliar, to make sure that somebody does not rush off with your bag never to be seen again. Most taxi drivers will usually volunteer to carry your bag for you. If they don't, change your taxi driver.

Remember, if you are going somewhere and the hotel has a laundry service, pack less and use the service. It will be more expensive but probably far less expensive than the damage you'll do to your back. The debilitation, the pain and time it will take to recover again could ruin your journey. Sensible planning can mean you take far fewer clothes, many of which you can put through the laundry system and some to wash in your hotel room.

A final note on travelling light. Toiletries tend to be heavy when added up – do you need to take so much? If you are going to a holiday destination or a business destination it is highly likely that they sell the items you need – so buy them at your destination. Many big hotels will have a small shop. They may be slightly more expensive – does that matter? The answer is probably no.

ACTION

- Start to walk as much as you can.

Chapter 12 – Tested approaches to ease the hassle of travel

- Aim to be as independent as soon as possible and only asking for assistance when you really need it.

- Be realistic with your travel expectations – you can probably do more than you think, and less than you would like.

- Be mindful of any kind of travel where you cannot get up and walk about.

- Travel light!

Chapter 13

Measuring, recording and monitoring changes

This may seem a little self indulgent but it is a valuable to measure a range of things that you do and feel.

Time to do things

If your mobility is restricted by back pain I would suggest that you choose some things that you do daily and start to record the time it takes to do them. Things such as:

- The time to get up and dressed each day.
- The time to get to the toilet once you are up from the usual place you sit at home.
- How long it takes to get to the kitchen.

I would suggest that you identify 3 or 4 key activities and use these as your base, your foundation, on which to build. Take an interest in how things are going and take it seriously too. This is not something to do occasionally or inconsistently – it is valuable information to record daily.

Also get some precision when timing yourself, or getting someone else to time you. You could use a portable kitchen timer or even a stop watch. This is not a race, just a means to record. A guess of 'about half an hour to get up' is not good enough – be precise and record it. If you are not at work you have the time to take these measurements and record them in a book in writing. If you are at work and are having some mobility difficulties you should also measure your performance so you can see how things change.

What you do

Review the things that you are doing. Is it just lying in bed and watching television or is it a whole range of things? Keep a list and start to see how life is going. It may be that you start to do less – establish why and have a focus to change things.

- If you are doing more how does this feel?
- Are those things that you are now doing, enabling you to develop a life that is returning to normal?
- Are you doing more things by yourself or do they include others who still need to help you?
- Are the things you are doing 'displacement activities' because the life you currently lead has little focus?
- Are they valuable things that are helping you regain your life?

Do get a clear view on your life – what you can do, what you cannot do, and what has changed?

A daily review

I also suggest that at the end of each day – perhaps shortly before you retire you spend a few minutes reviewing how your day has gone.

I found this an important conclusion to each day. Sometimes I felt elated at what I had achieved during the day. Some days I really felt 'flattened' as I have done so little, my pain levels were high and my mobility had decreased. Rather than end my day on a negative note, I would consider what had happened and consider if I had pushed myself too hard. Or had I pushed myself too hard the day before and this was the price I was paying. Or had I been too lazy. Getting downhearted achieved nothing although in the initial stages I was very hard on myself. Eventually I found it wiser, once I had reviewed my day to congratulate myself if it was a better day, and rule a line under each day whether good or not so good.

This is a crucial point – I began to realise that a poor day was usually before a breakthrough, I just didn't realise it at the time!

Level of pain

A critical part of understanding how you are improving in any form of rehabilitation is to measure where you have reached at any particular point. I suggest that you keep a daily log of the amount of pain or discomfort that you are experiencing. I also suggested that you choose one time during the day when you will be able to consistently evaluate the level of pain you are experiencing. It does not matter when in the day, just as long as it is a similar time.

Even if during the other parts of the day your pain levels have been very high, or very low, the measurement should be based on the level of pain you are suffering at the time you choose to record. Good times to measure are at a meal time or at a set time of the day when you would normally be in one place. I suggest that this could be at mid day or at five o clock both times are just before meal times or shortly after dinner say at 7 o'clock in the evening. It is important that the time is kept static and it is important that you make an assessment on how you feel at that particular time. The way to do this is to record your pain on a scale of 0 – 10 where 0 is no pain and 10 is extreme pain. It is difficult to grade the scale for everyone so just spend a little time yourself creating your own definitions associated with the level of pain. This may seem a little strange to do but the only person you are measuring against is yourself and the change of state that you will experience is your own. This is not a precise science so if the measurement is not specific it will not matter, you will develop a way of gauging things.

You may do this as a table with the date and the number between 0 – 10, or you could record on a graph like the one below. Keep it simple too.

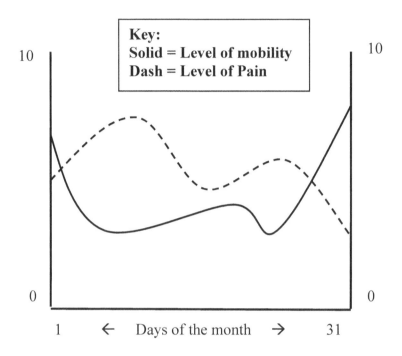

I created a scale with some definitions where I explained in a few words what each number meant. I refined this over time and as I got used to knowing how I felt and what pain really meant.

A second measurement that is worth taking, which ignores pain, is undertaking normal daily lifestyle tasks. This will include such things as:

- Getting up
- Showering/washing
- Getting dressed
- Cleaning teeth
- Ability to move around and walk

- Ability to undertake tasks around the house, such as:
    - Getting in and out of chairs
    - Preparing any food
    - Moving any small item around the house such as a magazine or book.

In fact anything you do with what you would consider normal activities in normal life.

The objective of a measurement is to understand how you are coping with the routine of daily living. As with the pain assessment above it is important, and valuable, to record each day your level of mobility and ability to cope with the daily routines of life.

Use a scale from 0 – 10 where 0 – is almost no mobility whatsoever to where 10 is the ability to maintain a normal life. I suggest you grade this scale yourself in a similar way as I have suggested with the pain scaling. Record your score at the same time as you record your pain score and do it every day. It can be done in the small table in your book or on the same graph so you have some comparison – do this by using two different colours.

Keep positive

During the recording of your pain levels and lifestyle movement you may notice in the early stages that your pain level increases and your mobility decreases. This is not unusual as you may be undertaking tasks for the first time in a long while and it is a natural reaction to increased activity.

This is no different from you being reasonably fit and exerting yourself with new exercise and suffering the aches that we all feel when we do this. As the example mentioned earlier in this book, if we go to the gym for the first time in a long while and push ourselves a bit too hard, we tend to ache for a couple of days afterwards. This is no different from what you are achieving by challenging yourself and undertaking activities to improve your long term back strength and health. Keep a watchful eye on this over a few days and you should see that the decreases in movement and increase in pain level will start to reverse. This is why it is important and a very valuable exercise to monitor your progress on a daily basis. Do not try and skip this part of the process, as your memory will never be good enough to establish the facts of how you were feeling day by day. One of the great challenges and pleasures associated with taking action to improve your back health is witnessing what is happening, because you are measuring the results.

As already mentioned, aim to record this information at a similar time each day. That way a pattern will start to form which can be viewed for days and weeks, and even months.

Do a new chart when the current one fills up. Even once you are back on your feet it is very useful to periodically fill in a chart for a week to reappraise how you are doing.

Other areas to consider measuring and recording are:

- Your flexibility.
    - How is it going?
    - What differences are you noticing?
    - Could you measure the distance you can bend with a tape measure?
- Your exercises.
    - The number of repetitions you have managed.
    - The range of exercises you are doing.
    - The frequency.
- Any activity you are choosing to time, such as:
    - Making a cup of tea.
    - Getting up in the morning.
    - The time it takes to get to the toilet.
- Your level of medication you are taking.
    - The types.
    - The amounts to ensure you are reducing over time.

I am sure there are more that you can think of too. My recommendation is to make sure you have a useful range that you are recording rather than try and measure everything.

Remember: You cannot manage what you do not measure.

ACTION

- Start your daily log.

- Commit to making notes each day.

- Measure a range of activities, write the results down and plot your progress.

- Set targets for yourself – ones that will stretch you but not defeat you.

- Create a pain and mobility graph and complete daily.

- Keep positive!

Chapter 14

Family, friends, neighbours: Take the right approach

Family, friends and neighbours are our support and lifeline especially in the beginning of back based problems. Many of the things that we can no longer do they can do on our behalf and they can offer major support at very difficult times.

My standing recommendation is always to ask when you are really struggling and be explicit so it is clear what you want doing. There is nothing worse for someone to find what they have done in good faith is not what was really needed. Also if you need a big favour still be explicit. Don't try and wrap it up in smaller things hoping that you can extend the request. Most people are delighted to help, they just need to know what is required. There is nothing worse than thinking that you are running a 30 minute errand to still find yourself tied up 4 hours later. If the original request asked for 4 hours it is probable that the person would have made arrangements so they could help.

The reaction from most people and especially caring family is to be massively supportive and look after most of your needs. I would stress that there is a real danger of you being "smothered" which will delay your short, medium and long term recovery. Their very kindness will actually slow the recovery process. This may seem quite heartless to refuse help when it is offered but it is absolutely critical that you are always stretching to look after yourself as much as possible. I will stress – it is your job to make sure that you are not being slowed down through kindness and love.

Examples of what family and friends can do that will really help in the early stages of your back problem.

- Driving you to critical appointments.
- Running errands which you cannot currently manage.
- Fetching and carrying heavy and bulky objects.
- Re arranging furniture at your request.
- Telephoning and speaking to wider circles of your family and friends so they know what is going on – a good idea is to create a 'buddy' system where one person may call 3 other people, and they in turn will call a further 3 people. This saves you, or another person spending hours on the phone. None of you need to and don't use it as an excuse to do nothing!

Examples of what family and friends will do that will delay your recovery:

- Bringing you chocolates, cakes and comforting treats.
- Bringing you white grapes.
- Cooking all your meals.
- Making you drinks.
- Turning the television on.
- Being so helpful that you lose any independence.
- Constantly telephoning, texting or expecting you to be on social media.
- Not being encouraging enough to let you make your own mistakes and push yourself. You need 'tough love'.

This may seem a little "cold" and also may burden you with tasks that are really painful to do. Remember, all of this is part of your recovery training program. Having to get up and turn the television on and off is an exercise in itself. Having to prepare and cook your meals gets you ready for a life where you are self sufficient again.

It is your responsibility to consider your family and friends as people that you really value. Only ask them to do things for you that you can genuinely not do yourself.

Celebrate and show the pleasure of each additional task you are undertaking as an indication of you returning to better health. Share with people who are close, the trials and tribulations of what you are going through but do not frighten them with every last gory detail of your suffering. Or bore everyone with your constant talking about yourself.

Keep a wary eye out to establish if you possibly ask too much from them.

A few tips:

- Don't say 'sorry' 20 times a day – if you are genuinely having a problem people do understand.
- Don't say 'thank you' 20 times a day either – it's value as a currency dies. Say it when you mean it and when it has some weight behind it because the person has gone the extra mile.
- Do thank people though.
- Try and avoid being miserable.
- In fact aim to be upbeat.
- Also don't become a bore with your problems.

People who look after you

Consider and appreciate them. It may not be easy but it is a vital part of showing respect for yourself and respect for others.

They need a life too so do encourage them to leave you alone and do something for themselves. This is especially important for people who live with you. If they have stopped hobbies or other activities, encourage them to get involved again. Do your utmost not to be a drain on them otherwise they will become bored and boring as there will be too little to talk about, too little to share and they will feel as if their lives are on hold as well.

At worst they will start to resent you being a drain on them, they will despair of you if you don't take control of your situation. Most will get annoyed if they cannot see you trying to get better. You have a health issue, not them.

Yes, so tough love but well needed for the sanity of all concerned. **And all too frequently overlooked.**

Remember you have a responsibility – to get as well as you can as fast as you can. So what are you doing next?

ACTION

- Ask for help when you need it but be honest and realistic with your requests.

- Set the ground rule with people who visit with 'treats' and too much support.

- Don't become a bore with your 'problem'. Keep up beat and interested in others too.

- Take action to show you are determined to get better.

- Appreciate others.

- Don't 'whinge'.

Chapter 15

How to be effective and comfortable at work

First things first

The first thing to establish is 'am I likely to be back at work soon?' It is often very difficult to establish this but it is vital to think this through.

Sometimes our problem will mean that we can go to work, albeit it may be a little draining and painful. Sometimes it is clear that for the next few days or possibly weeks we will not be able to attend. Be honest with your employer and be respectful too. I obviously don't know what the reaction of your employer will be although most are reasonable people and will try and be supportive of your needs.

When I had my major episode it meant that there was no way I could work. There wasn't the remotest chance of getting to work, being useful if I had got there, or even doing anything from home. Fortunately I had a very sensible employer who realised I was ill and not someone who normally took time off so they knew I had a problem. I was office-based and travelled extensively but certainly not doing heavy labour such as building work or lifting heavy loads. If that had been the case, I would have had to ensure that I was fit enough to be useful before I could return. Initially I was thinking about what I could do as soon as possible that would re-engage with my world or work – this was a totally unrealistic attitude and I needed to accept that I had a major problem and that I had to get better first. Until I was somewhat better I was of no use to my employer.

At this point **I realised that my 'new job' was to get better**. I had to take time out to ensure that I looked after myself. My tendency was to think that I've got to try and do some work. What tends to happen if you do try and work is whatever you do, you do poorly, with the consequence that you feel that you have let the staff or the team around you down. You also feel you have let yourself down too.

Firstly, focus on getting better.

Secondly, if you're lucky to have a generous employer that pays for some time off sick you have a genuine commitment to acknowledge that you are being paid to get well.

Anything you can do to get better is what you've got to do. Show respect for what your employer is doing for you while you're ill. This was the attitude I took.

I fortunately didn't end up in hospital but felt massively guilty about being away from work, letting my colleagues down. Once I realised that there was nothing I could do that would really help – I was unable to take sensible phone calls, not able to make good and fully informed decisions on things, certainly not able to write any decent material for my colleagues to work with, completely useless to my world of work – my focus changed. Changed to getting back to fitness, getting back to work.

Make sure your focus is on getting fit and back to work.
Some people will not take their responsibility to their employer seriously which I think is wrong.

The world does not owe us a living and nor does any employer owe us a livelihood – tough but true.

Doing nothing and stewing in my own juice was not an option. I wanted to be fit again. I wanted to get back to work. That became my mantra and my focus. It should be yours.

Attitude of mind

While you're off work it is a great opportunity to reassess what you do. Think about what you do at work and the impact this has on you. Determine what you need to do to get back to work and whether this is achievable.

Ask yourself the question 'Is the work I'm doing helping or hindering my physiology, and is this likely to cause me a problem in the future?'

I didn't want to change my job because I enjoyed it enormously, so I thought about what my job entailed. Forgetting the skills required to do the detail of my job but looking at my work pattern it revolved around:

- Sitting in a car.
- Driving between clients.
  - Sometimes in traffic, sometimes on quiet roads.
  - Some short journeys and some long ones too.
- Sitting at a desk.
- Working on a computer at work and at home.
- Standing up and speaking or presenting.
- Working long hours.
- Being punctual for appointments.

The key things I did were very clear.

- I sat at a desk.
- Sat in a car to drive, make notes or speak to people by phone.
- Stood up and spoke.

The next question was straight forward, 'How can I make sure that I'm fit to sit at a desk, fit to drive a car, fit to stand and speak?'

That became my focus – getting fit to do these things again and understanding what aspects of my work (or lifestyle) had caused my problem in the first place.

The majority of what I did at work was similar to how I normally live at home. Drive around, stand up and talk to people and sit at a table or sit on the sofa.

If I could get well at home I could transfer that to my workplace. The approaches to getting better I have covered throughout this book apply equally well at work too. So I considered all aspects of my new regime:

- How could I ensure that I ate well at work?
- How could I drink more water?
- How could I avoid coffee and tea?
- During the day I would need to stretch – how could I make that work?
- I would need to do some exercises – how could I do them at work?
- I needed to avoid getting stressed and take action if I did.
- I would need to look at the furniture where I worked for long periods of time.
- When I went to see clients or visit other parts of our organisation how would I utilise the furniture I would have to use?
- Was my briefcase too full and heavy and if so how would I carrying papers and materials?
- The list goes on....

We can all make these changes. As examples:

1. I couldn't sit down for any length of time at all at work because it was so uncomfortable, so I found a place and told people I was disappearing where I could lie on the floor for five minutes and have a good stretch. It got rather amusing, people used to accept that. Once I'd sorted those

sorts of things out it was accepted that in my recovery period I would be lying on the floor periodically or I would be standing up stretching. For some meetings I would stand, this had the benefit that it made the meetings shorter! At some larger meetings that were going to last a longer time I would make sure that I sat somewhere I could stand without causing too much disruption. For other meetings I arranged to attend only for the agenda item that I was needed for. These actions had the benefit that it saved time and made me more focussed. Attributes of good time management anyway!

2. I also got used to carrying herbal tea, as it was far less common than it is today. It became known as 'Peter's funny tea' and solved the coffee and tea issue.

3. I have mentioned elsewhere in this book that it is recommended that you should never sit in a car longer than two hours at a time. Preferably no longer than 90 minutes no matter how good the car is and how good a driver you are. To this day that is something that I do – 90 minutes then I'm looking for a service station. I had a quality German car which flashed a warning up at 2 hours – they did this for a reason and I found it invaluable to make me stop on the odd occasion I forgot my 90 minute rule. It worked then and still works now.

4. The same applies at a desk. I didn't sit at a desk for hours on end. I got up and did a few stretches, some other tasks that got me moving about. Making sure that they were linked to what I was working on – there's so much I could do. I was not disrespectful to my employer and colleagues, I was paid to work – but it was and is a way I ensured that I regained my self-respect and belief in myself.

I became very effective in the world of work and in many ways far better than I had before. A great bonus!

For anyone whose work is demanding physically it is important to consider getting fit enough to continue to undertake the work for which they have been trained. After a period off work muscles quickly become weak through the lack of use so it is important to start to get fit again using a good exercise regime. There are many exercises that can be undertaken that will strengthen 'core muscles'. These are the muscles that protect the spine and also give the foundation for good fitness. In addition, if the work is quite strenuous, additional exercises may well be needed. Most gyms have fitness instructors – some are excellent and will help you develop a good regime of exercise. Some are less good so, as I have frequently mentioned throughout this book, take personal responsibility and ownership. Most people can get fit enough to return to active work.

If it is clear that this is not the case it is wise to discuss things with your employer – most are very sensible and sensitive and will help people return to work. Having good dialogue is crucial so you can raise concerns and it is better to take charge of your situation rather than let things unfold where you have less control. As a general statement most employers are hugely supportive about trying to ensure that a valued employee returns to work at an early opportunity. If it is clear that the type of work will have to change to accommodate your physical problems many an employer will consider relocating you in a different part of the business, and in some cases re-training you too.

So ask yourself these two questions:

1. Is my employer likely to listen and care about my situation so I can have a good conversation and feel that they care?

2. Am I respected well enough as an employee to be considered for redeployment in my organisation?

If the answer to either question is no, start to think about what you may have done to your employer that you may need to change when you get back. Also what you may need to do is make sure they do value you rather than just see you as a pair of hands to do some work. Also really think about the type of work you are doing – is this what you want to carry on doing?

Often major incidents in our life are great opportunities to take stock and review what we want to do. I know I found the whole experience very focussing and really did use the time I was not at work to really think through my future in a very positive way.

At this time it is also a good idea to think wider than your world of work. I am not unrealistic enough to think that life and changes are easy. They are not, but if you have had a health issue such as your back pain now may be a forced opportunity to review your lifestyle.

- Are you leading the life that is appropriate for maintaining good quality health?
- Your lifestyle got you to where you are now – is this where you want to be?
- If you want to make changes what are they?

Review your lifestyle by going through every chapter of this book. We have covered a wide range of issues that are all areas that can help cure your back pain.

When I reviewed my lifestyle I had to make some clear changes. I knew what I was like with my work. As I enjoyed what I did and liked the challenge I worked very hard. I was like a light switch, I was either on or off – I could not imagine giving less than 100% and needed to reconsider the life I was leading. That is why I decided to leave my job in corporate life and set up my own business – it was a lifestyle choice.

I also knew that I needed to remain active and alter the way I lived my life. When I spoke to my medical consultant his diagnosis was very simple, **"Continue to remain fit and have an**

active life and you'll be one of the fittest 80 year olds around. Stop and you will soon have a back problem which means that you'll be unable to walk in later life." I had a very simple choice.

I do have a lifestyle that incorporates activities which I enjoy. Importantly I integrate them into my normal daily life so that they're not 'add on extras'. Do look at your lifestyle and everything else around you and consider – is the lifestyle I'm leading right for the type of health I want for my future? A big question and one I am sure you know the answer to!

If your work is mostly desk bound it is crucial to make sure that you take every opportunity to look after your back health.

As mentioned before, make sure you have what is called a 'workplace assessment', which establishes the height of the desk, the type of chair you're sitting at, and, if you are using a computer, to make sure the computer is positioned in the right place. This will ensure from a health and safety point of view that you've got exactly the right working conditions that you need. A typical office chair is usually fine, but all too often they are an old piece of furniture, or something you've inherited, that is not right for you. Sometimes it has past the end of its useful life. If this is the case consider getting something that is right for you.

I mentioned I was very heavily desk and car bound with my work. When I returned to work I had a proper work place assessment undertaken. I was a little sceptical as to why I needed this although I went along with the idea. I found it amazing to reconsider my workplace and how I had taken it for granted. I was well looked after before and the furniture was good, but it was not quite right for me. I have mentioned some of the details in the furniture section but it is worth repeating here, as this is one of the areas where, in my view, it is vital to invest some time and get everything right. Initially anything feels uncomfortable and seems to be a compromise. Get things right and it will all help with your recovery, get it wrong and it will probably make your problem worse.

This has been touched on in chapter 11, but it is well worth covering again for the area of work. The standard size desk is 29 inches (approximately 73 centimetres) tall. The reason it's 29 inches is because it fits through a door, a standard British door. It's not because it's the best height to work at. And certainly, as we as a population are becoming taller, for many people that is too low. I am 6ft tall and my current desk is 31 ½ inches (80 centimetres) tall so it's 2 ½ inches (approximately 6 centimetres) more than a traditional desk. Even if you are also 6ft tall you may need a different height, as your back:leg ratio may be different. People who are less tall may need something a little lower. Likewise taller people may need something a little higher. One size definitely does not fit all.

Importantly, the chair is a critical part of the whole and will also need to match your desk. If your desk works for your height it may be as simple as having a chair that is height adjustable and putting a foot rest under your feet to give you support. If your desk does need its height increased the chair will need to be correspondingly higher to. This is where a fully adjustable chair is valuable so don't overlook this fact.

The ideal seat is where the horizontal part is slightly sloping forward. The edge where your knees are is lower than where your bottom is seated. You might think it is completely odd and uncomfortable, but it is by far the best way to sit. When I returned to work I had a new chair, which was adjusted just for me, to ensure that I could sit on it comfortably. It was a revelation to have a chair measured and adjusted to fit me properly and I have no hesitation in saying it was a significant and positive part of my rehabilitation. They key features where:

- Adjustable height.
- Arms to rest my elbows when I was working at my desk or on my computer.

- An adjustable seat so I could tilt the horizontal part forward to get my knees lower than my bottom.
- A good shaped back which gave me support, even when I was working and the seat was tilted forward.

Take your seating very seriously. This extends to the car, especially if you are spending significant periods driving, or even sitting in a car as a passenger.

Check the car seats. Check the layout.

These are some areas to consider:

- Check where the steering wheel is positioned.
  - o This may seem like a strange statement but some steering wheels are not quite central so your arms, when holding the wheel are not uniform and straight
- Is there rake and reach adjustment?
  - o This is not always important but it does provide opportunities to get a perfect sitting position
- Are the pedals central?
  - o This is a valuable area to check. I noticed on one car specifically that the pedals were offset, so when you sit you are sitting slightly twisted. This really surprised me, so by sitting and checking this out before you drive off you may notice that to depress the pedals that you are not always 'square on'. This is not confined to small cheap cars, the ones I have noticed most are expensive mid range executive cars. Cars that are driven by many people covering considerable distances each year. I am sure this is storing up all kinds of problems for the drivers – horrifying! Check this area out!
- The height of the seat.
  - o Are you going to be struggling to get down or up to the seat to sit in the vehicle? When in the

vehicle can you adjust the seat so you are high enough to see out comfortably, or low enough?

- Is the door heavy to open and close?
  - o Consider the strain this may place on you and just check that you feel comfortable with the weight from both the outside and once you are seated and need to close and open the door from within.
- Is the boot (trunk) lid heavy to lift and the right height for you?
  - o This could be an issue if it is needed to be lifted often and ensure it is not too high to reach easily or too low to feel comfortable.
- Are the doors big?
  - o If you park frequently in tight spaces it may not be easy to get out of the vehicle. Where there are two doors rather than four, they tend to be longer and make the problem worse.
- Is the height of the door frame comfortable?
  - o It needs to be high enough to get in and out without having to struggle and bend your neck.
- Is there sufficient head room?
  - o Some cars you may find the roof of the car is too low so your head brushes the roof lining – subconsciously you will keep moving your head and this may cause neck or shoulder problems. I have sat in many cars where my head is close to the roof and whilst fairly tall I am not excessively so.
- Does the seat back have rake adjustment?
  - o You should not be lying back, nor sitting too bolt upright. Some adjustment is useful to make the position better for you. Make sure the adjusting control is easy to use.
- Do the controls fall easily to hand?
  - o Make sure you do not have to constantly reach for any that you may use regularly.
- Are the rear view mirrors well placed?

- o You need to see them without having to strain yourself.
- Do the wipers clear enough screen?
    - o When it is raining or the screen is dirty ensure you have a clear line of sight. Many cars on UK roads are designed for left hand drive, not right hand drive, and the 'sweep pattern' leaves a blind spot in the right hand side of the screen which causes you to slightly lean to the left or move more often than is needed.
- Is the suspension too firm?
    - o Many manufacturers love the large wheels and sports suspension. This tends to be firmer than the standard set up and can make the ride especially harsh if the roads are poor quality as they are in much of the UK after a bad winter.
- Do you carry samples or items in the boot regularly?
    - o Ensure they will be easy to get out of the boot (trunk).
- Is there sufficient space to put any bags or brief cases without having to strain?
- If you will need to lift the bonnet (hood) often, check you can reach the 'pull' inside the vehicle and lift the bonnet – it may be awkward, heavy or both.
    - o You may need to top up the oil or screen wash frequently. Can you get help when needed?

I certainly found from driving the occasional commercial vehicle that there's a dramatically wider range of seat movements than there is in your average family car. Primarily because they're designed for people who drive for a living and spend most of their day on the road.

Use the adjustments that are there. Don't make do. It is your back health at stake.

An interesting exercise to do is to look at how other people sit in their vehicles. Do this when you are at the traffic light and you will be amazed how some people sit – it is clear they are storing up trouble for later in life. There are those who lie back and peer over the wheel, those whose seat is heavily reclined but they sit forward with little of the seat in contact with their back, those who sit bolt upright, and so the list goes on – do have a look and consider how you sit, you may realise that you should be sitting better than you are!

If you're reading this as someone who is a member of a family of someone who has a back problem and you are fit, in your mid 20s you might think this is all ridiculous. You feel fine and this is all overplayed. I can guarantee over the years in front, if you continue to have bad posture and a poor attitude to looking after yourself when sitting, at some point in the future you will have a back problem.

Now spend some time considering:

- What are your key elements of work?

- What do you need to change?

ACTION

- Show respect and openness with your employer.

- Focus on getting better so you can get back to work.

- Review what your role at work entails and determine if anything will need to change.

- Ensure that you do not sit for prolonged periods of time.

- Organise the changes that are needed.

Chapter 16

Tips for a better night of sleep

Your aim is to take no sleeping tablets. Period. There should be no need. There is a risk if you do take strong medication because you will not be aware of your body and the stresses and strains it is experiencing which may exacerbate your problem if you are 'dead to the world'.

I have never taken any sleeping tablets even when the pain was dreadful. My guess is you don't need to either. If your medical practitioner has prescribed medication, is that because you have 'laid it on thick' and insisted or because you have a different medical complaint that warrants them? Be brutally honest.

If you are currently on medication you may well have to come off slowly to avoid the withdrawal symptoms and will need to involve your medical practitioner with this too. Seek proper advice, don't just stop.

I would also add that the section on food and drink did mention that an occasional relaxing drink is fine. If you are having a large stiff drink every night to help you get to sleep you have missed the point! If you are mixing this with medication.........!!

I am being deliberately tough on this as I have heard so many people say, 'you don't understand how bad it is'. **I DO.** That is why I can give you this advice.

When and where to sleep

This is quite simple. Sleep in bed, at night.

Do not fall asleep in a chair. These are a few reasons why not:

- Your posture will be dreadful.

- You will probably ache when you wake up.
- Your breathing will be poor meaning your blood will not get the oxygen it needs.
- If you sleep during the day you will be less likely to sleep at night.
- If you have friends or family in the room it is rude.

If you feel that you need a doze, ask yourself why. Is it because you have over eaten, or had an alcoholic drink? If either is the case perhaps the message is to eat less and avoid alcohol.

Unless you are a shift worker the time and place to sleep is at night and in bed. Aim to get into a routine, where you get up at a reasonable time in the morning and you retire at a reasonable time too.

During the day you should be undertaking your exercises and other activities. If you are in a lot of pain these activities will drain you and make you tired. In an odd way that is one of their purposes, to use your body so that you are naturally tired and will sleep.

If you are not active at all during the day you need to start getting active and doing something that has been covered in earlier chapters. If you are doing nothing, be firm with yourself – is it because others won't let you do anything so they are smothering you in kindness or is it because you are avoiding doing things? It is one or the other. You know the answer and whatever it is it needs to change.

How to get comfortable in bed

It may not be possible but if you can, it is wiser to have a bed to yourself – certainly in the early recovery stages. Take bed time seriously and aim to make it a relaxing and pleasurable time too. Here is a range of things to do to help you get comfortable in bed and also to help you to sleep. These are based on my experience and include:

- Make sure your bed is regularly changed so it is fresh and clean.
- Ensure that there is no crunched up undercover to make it uncomfortable.
- A fitted sheet is best as it is less likely to come adrift if you toss and turn.
- A duvet is easier to manage than sheets and a blanket and get less twisted and uncomfortable. Have a light one in the summer and a heavier one in winter.
- Use bed socks if it is cold.
- Night clothes are a personal choice – they keep you warm, dignified and clean. They can twist and turn and get uncomfortable.
- If you have not done your exercises earlier in the evening do them before you shower.
- Have a shower before you retire so you are clean and fresh.
- Use a lavender gel in the shower, as it will relax you.
- A bath, if you can get in and out, is even more relaxing – also use lavender oil or bath gel to relax you, not too much though.
- Use one pillow for your head.
- Have two other pillows in reach – one to support your back and....
- If you are more comfortable on your side put a pillow between your knees, either the central part that is full of the filling or the outer edge, which is less thick.
- Open the window to let in some fresh air if you can. Not too wide in case it rains. If you live in a country where it is hot and you have air conditioning this does not apply, likewise if it is subzero. Also don't open the window if it lets in bugs, especially if they bite. Keep the window closed if it is very noisy.
- Have a bedside light with the on/off switch in easy reach.
- Have a glass or plastic bottle of water in easy reach.
- Find a good book that you enjoy. Read a chapter before you try and go to sleep.

- Have a small pad of 'post-it' notes and a pencil to hand. Anything you think of during the night write down.
- If you are so inclined have a fury stuffed friend – not a live pet.
- Go to bed and get up at a reasonable time.
- Have a small alarm clock and set it at a reasonable time so you can get up and not waste the day.
- Do not treat your bed as a day bed.
- Relax.

Don't be concerned about enjoying your bed. It should be a haven where you can sleep and restore your strength. If you have had a day where you have been busy doing the right things to get better you should value time here. Do not become lazy and **do set yourself a target that you will get up at a sensible time whether you have slept or not**. I will guarantee if you use the excuse that you have not slept and stay in bed till noon, you will have another night in front of you when you will not sleep.

ACTION

- Avoid sleeping tablets and if you are on these set yourself a target to reduce and then eliminate them. Discuss with your medical practitioner.

- Stop dozing during the day.

- Only sleep in bed and at night (unless your work demands dictate otherwise).

- Make your bedroom a haven for relaxation with everything near at hand that you need.

- Get up at a sensible time every day.

Chapter 17

Setting goals and having focus

Have a focus!

One of the key things that I know helped me solve my back problem was having focus – and having a reason. Once I realised I had a major problem and it was not going to be a few pills and a week off work that would sort me out I took control of the situation. I developed a clear set of goals and started to measure my progress. The chapter on measuring how you are doing is a critical part of recording the knowledge of what works, and what does not. This was a major motivator to look and see the steps I was taking. Each small achievement would have been lost without me recording them. And recording them with my focus in mind.

Creating and then maintaining your focus is a significant part of your recovery. For me it was a crucial part of the whole of my recovery process.

Now some questions to help you get your focus:

- What is your focus?
- What is your first goal?
- What is your objective that you are aiming to achieve?
- What could be the first step?

As an example, my first objective was to live a moderately normal life. My definition of moderately normal at that time was where I could:

- Do most basic domestic household activities.
- Drive a car.
- Walk a reasonable distance to get things.
- Do my own basic shopping.

Nothing wildly exciting but these were going to be major achievements for me. Quite simply a life where there was a degree of normality and independence.

That was my first focus. To achieve that I had to break things down into much smaller tasks. Tasks such as:

- What were the domestic activities?
- What did I need to do so I could drive?
- What was the distance I needed to be confident to walk so I could get out?
- Where could I shop?
- How much shopping could I carry?
- Could I deal with a supermarket trolley?

The next focus was to return to being a fully functioning adult. My definition included:

- Back to work properly.
- Walking on the hills if I wanted to.
- Socialising.
- Living most of my life as it was before.
- Adjusting parts of my life that I had decided I wanted to change.
- Maintaining my overall health and integrating my back care exercises into a daily routine.

The clarity for me was focusing on the small steps I need to take to get there. Then focusing on each of those steps in turn and determining what I had to do. Steps such as:

- What diet should I be following?
- What food should I be eating?
- Making sure I adhered to good diet and eating.
- What exercises should I be doing?
- Measuring what impact they were having.
- Focusing on flexibility and watching my development.

- Deciding on my activities around the house and setting a timetable.
- Reviewing what I was achieving and if I needed to do more.

I had a plan of action that I was thinking through to retain that focus.

These are some of the questions I kept asking myself to keep focused, to keep me moving forward. They may help you too:

- Is my posture good? Sitting or standing.
- Am I using the furniture well?
- Am I doing my exercises?
- When did I stretch last?
- Am I eating regularly and the right things?
- What time did I get up today?
  - o Was I late and if so why?
  - o If I was earlier is that now my new benchmark time?
- Am I drinking the right things?
- Am I drinking enough water?
- Am I getting the right level of support?
- Am I turning away the over-supportive people who are trying to do too much for me?
- Am I getting lazy?
- Am I watching too much TV?
- What have I done today that was a bigger challenge than yesterday?
- Where do I ache and why?
- Why don't I ache, have I not tried hard enough?
- ....and more.

You could add your own to the list too.

Do write down your thoughts and plan your actions – if you just think and don't write anything down your thoughts will get lost. If you think, then write, you can plan your action – and record the action you took.

People who plan on paper get results. People who plan in their mind procrastinate!

The one thing that people with major back problems, who are not at work have, is time. Therefore you have time to think things through, time to plan, time to think about what you're going to do the following day and what you need to do today. TIME TO TAKE ACTION.

People who say to me 'I don't have time to do the suggested exercises, and twice a day!' I would ask 'What else are you doing?' Watching television won't get you better. Talking to your friends won't get you better. Sitting around won't get you better either – my guess is that time is plentiful – so take action. People who say I don't find the time to do the exercises when they are much better have lost their focus and set themselves up for a relapse. You have choices.

Keeping a focus, both during and after the initial episode, is absolutely crucial. When you start to really get the whole ethos of what we're talking about well embedded in what you do, it will become a way of living. And therefore second nature. You get used to remembering every morning to do your exercises. Every evening you remember to do your exercises. It becomes something you naturally do. Most people have a bath or a shower before they go out in the morning to work, or at the end of the day when they come in from work. If somebody said to you stop washing you'd think it was unnatural. That's the way I feel with the exercises. That is the way you can feel with the focus you have on looking after your back.

I do stress that it does become second nature and you automatically consider what you do. It is a way of life where no one will guess that you have had a back problem. Yes, we will have lapses, we are only human!

As a final point in this section, do not become obsessed with your back problems. You can deal with it in a way that starts to be 'below the radar'. I would strongly suggest that you reengage with one of your hobbies or pastimes that have been left to one side. The very action of focussing on something else will help you too. It will also focus other people's attention away from your back problem as well.

What I am sharing is what I have learnt and a whole raft of things I have developed for looking after my back so I can live a completely normal, very active life.

They are things you can learn and use too. If you keep focused.

ACTION

- What is your focus (write it down and be specific)?

- Set the actions you are going to take.

- Make the time to do what you need to do – exercises, planning, setting the right steps, taking action, recording results.

- Check that you are taking action.

Chapter 18

Promises and pitfalls of alternative therapies

There are a significant variety of alternative therapies that can be considered. I believe taking a holistic approach to the treatment of your back problems is an excellent idea. I would strongly advise that you consider a number of these on your journey to improved health and see what works for you.

Whilst any decent medical practitioner and especially any decent practitioner of alternative therapies will want to help you recover, the ultimate responsibility is yours and yours alone.

Important Note

Be mindful of any service for which you are paying where treatment is carrying on for extended periods of time without an ongoing reduction of pain. There is the risk that a small minority may see your pain as an opportunity for their gain. Any practitioner who is seeing you on a very frequent basis for a very long period of time has not got your interest at heart – fact. The objective of any high quality practitioner either medical or alternative therapy is to speed your recovery and do themselves out of work because they have been successful in helping you to return to self sufficiency.

Some of the areas that you could consider are as follows:

- Physiotherapists
- Chiropractors
- Osteopaths
- Reflexologists

- Aromatherapists
- Massage therapists
- Sports injury therapists
- Acupuncture practitioners

This list is by no means exhaustive and covers only some of the ones I have tried.

Perhaps the most useful information I can impart is my own experience having tried many varieties and what has worked for me.

Physiotherapists

> I used a very experienced and respected physiotherapist on a periodic basis over a number of years. He was excellent and I tended to go and see him when I was in some pain and my back was twisted and out of shape. He would do a proper and detailed review of me by looking at my spine and the way the rest of my body looked – this was always a visual examination. He took detailed notes having asked me a range of questions about my health and habits as well as my guess as to what may have caused the episode I was seeing him about. Only then would he ask me to get on the couch or a chair before he would start to massage me for quite a period of time to loosen my muscles before he would manipulate me. I would have one or two session, sometimes a few more in a very bad case and them it would be months or a year or so before I would go back when I had a further problem.

> When I went to see him after my last, and major, problem he saw I was in a terrible state. He carefully examined me and said I had a major problem that was not treatable by physiotherapy. I admire to this day his honesty and awareness of my problem.

Chapter 18 – Promises and pitfalls of alternative therapies

Chiropractors

After the physiotherapist, it was suggested that I try a chiropractor who has a different approach to problems from a physiotherapist. I was recommended a very good one and saw him on a very regular basis over a period of a few weeks. I kept challenging why so frequently and why was the treatment showing no signs of help.

His diagnosis was I would never walk properly again and recommended I came back on a regular basis to stabilise things. I hobbled out and have not seen him since. I have also proved him wrong!

Osteopaths

They specialise in making sure that all of the bones in the body are structurally aligned and this is usually done by manipulation. Often after some massage of the soft tissue. I saw an osteopath and we decided that the problem I had was inappropriate for their treatment methods.

Reflexologists

This is where the main treatment is the application of pressure to parts of the feet and hands. I found it a strange and pleasant feeling, which helped with relaxation, but in the early stages of a major back problem I found little direct relief, although the indirect feeling was lovely for a short period of time.

Aromatherapists

They use aromatic oils to stimulate the body's senses and healing. It is a soft form of massage with, in my case, soothing smelling essential oils. I am not sure of the medical impact for major structural damage that I had but, and this is a lovely but, I fell asleep and woke up wonderfully rested at the end of the session.

Massage – undertaken in a spa

The massage is very pleasant and many spas will have this type of massage. I found it relieved some surface tension in my back albeit with little long term benefit. I would have a massage for pleasure and enjoy the relaxation not expecting major results.

Sports injury massage therapists

This type of massage is very different from the ones that are found in general spas. Usually you will find someone through a good sports centre or specialist sports ground or centre such as rugby, tennis, swimming or a gym. It is also called a 'deep tissue massage' and you need someone who has been well trained.

The first massage I had I could not believe the effort the person needed to exert to treat me. I also could not believe the impact it had on me. I did wriggle when he dug deep but he was aligning the muscle tissue to support the joints and bones in the correct way.

To this day I have a regular deep tissue massage and the therapist I use is brilliant. She has got used to my body and can quickly find the tight areas that need work. She takes a holistic approach and the deep massage covers most areas of my body. It still amazes me that a tight muscle in one part of my body can have a major impact on another part somewhere quite different. I find this a perfect complement to my exercises and lifestyle and is the only therapy I do have on a regular basis.

Acupuncture practitioners

The use of needles inserted into various pressure and focal points of your body help relieve tension and some pain. It is based on a Chinese medicine that goes back over thousands of years. I found the localisation was effective in reducing pain in specific areas, although I did not try it long enough to have the feeling that it would cure a structural problem with my spine, muscles and damaged soft tissue. Fascinating though!

Summary

As I mentioned at the start of this chapter I have tried other therapies too. There are many more that I have not tried. For me the deep tissue massage works and makes sense in the way it works – releasing tense and knotted muscle, making sure it is supporting your joints and ensuring that everything is correctly in its place, improving flexibility. The lady who treats me also adds in some other therapies that she has significant expertise in (including horse massage!). Importantly I have never felt that I am an expected part of her monthly pay cheque – something I can assure you I have found with some other therapists.

As I have said all along in this book, make your own choices and stay in control. I have found it is so easy to be drawn into things because you are in pain and will try anything if you have some money, and almost pay anything for the next and latest therapy hoping it is 'the one'. My final comment – tread carefully!

ACTION

- Consider some of the alternative therapies.

- Critically review any therapies that you have been having where there is no noticeable improvement. Especially ones where you have been attending for prolonged periods of time.

- With the knowledge you can develop about your body whilst relaxing, consider any new thoughts you have regarding your pain and help that could be valuable.

- What is your body telling you?

Chapter 19

Avoiding the vicious circle: Taking responsibility

I believe this is one of the most important chapters in the book.

I have personally felt a 'vicious circle' surrounding me, and being drawn under its spell when I have been suffering. I have seen so many people who are caught under the spell and don't even realise what has happened to them. As you have chosen to invest in this book I don't want you to fall under the spell too.

The main problem with being ill, or suffering with back problems, is that there is a tendency just to make do. This is not good enough. What will happen over a period of time is that a slow and nasty vicious circle will form. This may take weeks or months – where the less you aim to rectify the problem the more difficult it will be to either start or make progress. Slowly and surely the longer term prognosis for your back problem will be poor and you start to see no end. Changes will happen:

- You will start to be able to do less.
- You may start to put on weight.
- You certainly will become less fit.
- You become less mobile.
- You partake in fewer activities with friends, with family and for yourself.
- You start to do nothing.
- You start to get an element of dependency on other people and other things around you.
- You start to lose the ability to look after yourself.

Chapter 19 – Avoiding the vicious circle: Taking responsibility

No matter what point you have reached this **vicious circle needs to be broken**. It will require strong will power. You need to start to undertake lifestyle changes and the areas covered in this book will enable you to resolve many of the problems you currently have. Do take the courage to do something. And to start right now.

No matter how hard it is, if you stop doing anything, your body loses its muscle strength, so the capability to do very much starts to go too. If you stop using your mind because you are no longer at work and don't do anything to replace the stimulation you had, that will start to become dull too.

I remember many years ago when in was ill and did not do very much I started to really lose mental capability. This got to such a point that my wife brought me some interesting magazines and told me that I was losing my edge! I was fortunate, and realised what had started to happen through her kind action. I was becoming, what is called 'institutionalised'. Horrifying how quickly this can happen! Important that someone around you notices, and crucial for everyone's benefit, including your own, that you do something. I was young at the time and it does happen at all ages, and quicker than you will realise.

With much less social interaction, you start to find that your mind isn't as sharp. Your brain is just like another muscle, the more you use it the better it becomes. Or you end up in this vicious circle where you start do less and less.

Take note if you start to become forgetful, time seems to disappear, you become lazy, can't be bothered and everything is an effort.

Even if you take small steps to do something it will create a major difference compared with doing nothing. Encouraging yourself to do something will make a difference. Don't rely upon other people to do everything for you, be stubborn as doing things for yourself is vital. Each little thing is valuable.

Chapter 19 – Avoiding the vicious circle: Taking responsibility

Muscles start to deteriorate within 36 hours. This is a horrifying fact that from the second you start doing less than you did before you will start to lose muscle tone and muscle strength. If you don't do anything for weeks on end, you may find that you can barely walk. If you don't get out of bed you probably will not be able to walk. This may sound alarmist – I can assure you this is correct and will happen.

We know, or have heard of people, who are in bed for a period of time and find that when they get up they can barely walk. When they do start to walk it's so difficult because they have so little strength left. They get tired very quickly, haven't got the strength to climb the stairs easily, feel lightheaded and their balance is not very good.

1. Anything you can do to retain some muscle tone is going to be valuable. Even if you are sitting in a chair or lying in bed there are things that you can do. Clenching your fists, squeezing the muscles in your arms, curling your toes and, stretching your feet, tensing the muscles in your legs just to get some activity to retain some muscle tone. If you are sitting in a chair, and it has arms, just gently lift yourself up, even if you only get your body into tension it is actually helping your muscle tone.

   The key thing is to start doing something, even a little is far better than doing nothing. For the sake of your muscles, start doing something. It may hurt – just accept that's the case and do something. As I have said to many people the pain may be inevitable, but the suffering is optional! I am not trivialising your situation – start and set yourself targets, even if small, and then work towards them.

2. Next, start to think about what you are eating. It is so easy to eat simple food or cheap food that comes out of a cupboard or sweet food that feels and tastes good – don't! You will put on weight and give your body poor quality

fuel with which to repair itself. It is so easy to eat 'comfort' food because you are not feeling good about yourself – don't!

3. Avoid drinking sodas or fizzy drinks because they're easy. You will slowly start to put on weight because you are not burning off the calories. It may not be noticeable initially as the weight creeps on little by little. Remember if you are not doing anything active you don't need as many calories. Certainly not as much as you normally eat, so if you continue to eat the same you will put on weight.

4. Avoid 'treats' else they will become part of the vicious circle. Do you have the will power to not eat the presents people bring? Who else will eat them? Is there an expectation building if you thank them profusely? An expectation they may start to resent, as they feel taken for granted. My advice – if they are true friends have a good conversation with them. If you don't it will be more difficult later to break this vicious circle, I am sure you agree.

5. Avoid temptation. It is so easy eat that piece of chocolate, or cake, or that extra biscuit or two. Especially if you are watching television, a film or reading a book or magazine.

I may be labouring the point. This is for a reason. This vicious circle starts without us noticing, and can soon be a downward spiral. Slowly your weight starts to increase, and your body becomes less toned. Clothes no longer feel so comfortable so you start to dress a little bit more casually. Perhaps wearing tracksuit trousers and a loose t-shirt. Because they are comfortable you feel a little happier and less aware of what you are eating. The waistband is elastic so you don't notice the next few pounds. Now you feel a little less energetic. Men perhaps stop shaving because it is just a little too uncomfortable to stand for as long. A stubble chin soon becomes the normal. So what is the next area to slip?

Perhaps relationships in the home start to deteriorate because you are doing less, and seen to be caring less too. This becomes that vicious circle of deterioration and you end up so far in before you realise. Or you reach a stage where you don't even notice, which is even worse. You have to keep in touch with reality and not hide behind your problem. If you don't accept responsibility who else should!

Now stop and think. Are you in a vicious circle?

Did you answer that question truthfully?

Think:
- What state am I in?
- What should I be doing?
- What else could I do?
- Am I being fair to those around me?
- Have I taken responsibility for my health?
- Have I taken responsibility to get better?
- Am I being lazy?

The key point is to start to do something – and right now.

Even if you are bed ridden or confined to a chair for most of the day you can do something right now. So go on, put this book down for a few minutes and do something.

How did that feel?

- **Good** – well done! Now start to take action and record what state you are in and the progress you make.
- **Terrible** – well done for starting to do something. Your challenge is to realise that you have now just started the journey to better health. It is crucial you keep a record and measure your achievements. It is crucial to continue until it does not feel terrible. Remember one step at a time, and make those steps count.

Chapter 19 – Avoiding the vicious circle: Taking responsibility

You can do something to start to improve your muscle tone and to start to get your body active. Try it – it won't be comfortable, but try it anyway. Think about what you eat – think of that saying 'my body is a temple'. Don't put into your body things that you know should not be in there!

Think about your mind:

- What are you doing to stimulate that?
- Are you just reading the odd magazine that has got no intellectual challenge at all?
- Are you watching the latest episode of a soap opera?
- Are you a spectator of life or a player? Well, which is it truthfully?
- If you have children are you setting a great role model?
- Or are you doing nothing?
- We all have choices, what are yours saying about you?

All of these things are valuable to think about. Valuable to action. Respect your self esteem, set your own direction. Get something to start challenging your mind. Maybe start doing some puzzles, crosswords, Sudoku, to keep your mind active. Don't treat it as a one day exercise and forget. Try various different things, not just Sudoku and only Sudoku.

So start right now with some changes to stop you being entranced into that vicious circle.

Here are some thoughts especially if you are at home rather than work:
- With your mid morning drink (remember to avoid caffeine, and drinks with sugars) perhaps do a Sudoku puzzle.
- Later in the day try something else, maybe the crossword.
- Get involved with what you would like to eat and research recipes that are healthy.
- Consider what you could cook for yourself and others.

- While you are inactive or resting in between exercises or other activities deliberately take on a programme to enrich your life. Perhaps:
  - Learning a language so when you start travelling again you can gain more out of the experience.
  - Or reading about a sport you're interested in participating in.
  - Reading some literature that you are interested in, or enjoyed perhaps when at school.
  - If you have an interest in films read the books the films are based on – maybe before you see the film.
- Review what you watch on television and avoid having it on all the time.
- Study for something that would help your work and help you get better qualified.

There is so much that can be done, so do something.

Look at your physical appearance and ensure that you are caring how you look and how you care for yourself. Some questions to consider:

- Are you brushing your hair?
- Are you cleaning your teeth properly?
- Have you shaved or groomed your beard (if a man).
- Do you dress tidily?
- Are your shoes clean?
- Are you wearing clean clothes every day?
- Are they pressed and ironed?
- If not, why not? And don't use other people as the excuse!

If you live by yourself, yes it's tough, but most houses have an automatic washing machine so you haven't got to manually wash your clothes. Treat this as part of your journey to self sufficiency.

- Put the washing in the washing machine. That is one challenge for the day, which is great.
- The next challenge during the same day is to hang it on a clothes airer. If it's difficult to put the airer up ask someone to do it for you but put the washing on yourself.
- When it's dry take it off and sort it.
- If it needs ironing, and you are not at work and don't normally iron now is good time to learn. The success of ironing one shirt, and it may only be one shirt, is amazing. Remember that one shirt might be for the following day when you would look that little bit smarter than you currently do.

These small things really make a difference to your self esteem. So often I have seen people who, when they have a problem medically, allow themselves to lower their standards, and in some extreme cases, almost enjoy not getting better. They self-talk themselves into not getting better, with the consequence that they stop doing anything.

- They start eating the wrong foods.
- They don't exercise.
- They watch rubbish television day in, day out.
- They don't read anything.
- They slowly start to vegetate.
- They become a less interesting person.
- Their friends and families are less interested in seeing them because the conversation is so poor.

This is not you!

So what are you going to do to avoid or break out of that vicious circle and start on your journey of recovery?

Remember – everyone, and I repeat this; **everyone** has the opportunity to improve. Start now!

ACTION

- Is your pain due to inactivity and possible laziness? (Don't get defensive – no offence is meant.)

- Step back and consider if you may have been drawn into this vicious circle.

- Start to get active by doing small tasks that then build to larger ones.

- Start to do something to create muscle strength.

- Start to do something to keep 'mind strength'.

- Keep your standards high.

Chapter 20

Medical opinion and working with your practitioner

Some medical practitioners are brilliant at understanding back based problems, many are far less knowledgeable. Inevitably after initial investigations by a general medical practitioner for extreme cases you may have been referred to a specialist medical adviser. Increasingly there is a desire to avoid surgery – which is good. Do be aware that if you are being referred to an orthopaedic surgeon, neurosurgeon or general surgeon their main skill set for which they have trained is surgery. This does not mean that they will always want to operate but certainly it will be a significant bleep on their radar.

Unless you have significant symptoms that warrant immediate surgical intervention, be very cautious. Many people who undergo surgery and gain short term relief can have relapses later in life. There is a significant school of thought that surgical intervention is not always the best treatment.

Even if you have had surgery it is not always a cure for life. I have known people who many years later have major relapses and end up with a second surgical procedure. This also carries the risk of a further general anaesthetic too and is not always the end to their problem.

We all know someone or have heard of someone who is unfit, overweight, smokes like a chimney, drinks like a fish and who has never had any ill health problems. Also the reverse is true and we know people who are fit, eat sensibly, don't smoke or drink and have major health issues. There seems to be no rhyme or reason.

Overwhelming medical evidence indicates that it is better to have respect for our bodies and exercise, eat sensibly, don't smoke, and drink in moderation – also common sense tells us that this is probably the best way to live too. The problem is that common sense is anything but common practise! I have aimed in other chapters to cover many aspects that all form a jigsaw. A jigsaw of creating an excellent opportunity for you to be fit and well with a great healthy back that causes you no further problems.

My first major back problem was back in 1984 when I had what was thought to be two prolapsed discs. I received good advice and support from my general practitioner and was eventually refereed to an orthopaedic surgeon. After an X-Ray he refused to operate as he thought the risk of permanent damage was too great. I ended up being encased in plaster from my waist to my chest for many weeks – not a pleasant experience especially as it was in the summer heat too.

My back became very weak due to the encasement and after it was taken off I had a relapse because my muscles were so weak. Not a good time in my life. Through careful living and some exercise I got back on my feet. I had a further comparatively minor relapse in 1991, and again, no surgery and back to a near normal life. It was some years later when I had my 'big one' when I was a real mess. Medical knowledge had moved on but back surgery was still a common place treatment – and it still is to this day. I took a very strong view, as I believed surgery would not solve my problems, as my back was in such a mess. There was talk of fusion of the vertebrae, metal reinforcement of my spine and other such things.

Fortunately I undertook a considerable amount of research whilst the investigations were being made and decided that an alternative approach was my way through. I was fortunate that my general practitioners were open-minded. The neurosurgeon I found was brilliant and NO I have not had surgery – he clearly told me at the outset that the vast majority of back surgery was not needed. I am in no position to challenge that but he was a massively experienced consultant who had trained to be a surgeon

– and wherever he could, he did not operate. Interesting, I am sure you agree! I now enjoy excellent health and have a back that is no longer a restraining influence on anything I do.

I am aware that other people have been guided through a medical maze. Many on strong medication. Many not able to work. Many having undergone surgery that has not been as successful as hoped. Many living a very inactive life. Many with dependency on those who are near. Yes, there are also cases where a full recovery has been possible.

I hope that you are tenacious enough to realise that this book provides you with an alternative. I cannot promise the same result I had. I am certain that if you have a back problem and follow the areas we have covered in this book you will be in far better health and more active than you currently are.

Take medical advice, listen to what is proposed. Question what is diagnosed.

Question the reason for any medication that is prescribed so you know:

- What it does.
- Why you are being prescribed this medication.
- Are there alternatives?
- Any likely side effects.
- The length of time you are taking the medication.
- Any effects when you stop taking it (if, indeed you start).
- Is it because the medical practitioner has misunderstood you?

Take ownership of your problem – do not abdicate your health care to anyone, work in partnership and take action to help yourself.
I will stress, work in partnership with your medical advisor and keep them informed. They are valuable people and will usually

respond well if they see you are really trying to get back to full health.

This book is full of advice and is totally based on what worked for me ~ you now have a choice.

ACTION

- Take responsibility and work with your medical practitioner.

- Question any indication that surgery is required.

- Discuss the reason behind any medication you need to take and crucially any the date it should be reviewed and cease.

- Take responsibility and importantly – action.

Final Comment

This book has covered a wide range of areas and I am sure it is not exhaustive by any means. There will be things that I take for granted that I have forgotten to mention. There will be things that you will develop that will also make a positive difference.

I do stress that taking action will help make that difference. Just reading this book is not enough – **action is key**.

And a crucial point is to become what I have termed:

'Back Wise'

Make a concerted effort to bring to your conscious mind that which you normally leave to the less conscious. That way, over time, you will start to become more aware of your back health and indeed start to become 'back wise' yourself.

My best wishes for your journey.

More information will be available at the following website:

www.TheBackChampion.com

Acknowledgements

The genesis of this book was developed at a business event on a grey November day. The reason I was sharing my story at the event was because an elbow encouraged me to stand up and speak. That elbow belongs to Yvette Nevrkla – as an author yourself your inspiration is valued beyond price.

The event I refer to was run by Neil Asher, a serial entrepreneur, whose post event letter included the comment: *"Peter's story brought a tear to my eye."* Thank you Neil for your support and encouragement.

As always getting a book into print is an effort involving many people. The guidance of my mentor Stephanie Hale has been invaluable. She is an author herself and helps others write, sell and promote their books through The Oxford Literacy Consultancy – I would recommend her to anyone who wishes to get their book to market.

There are also many other people who have travelled this journey with me – far too many to mention individually. They include loving and kind parents, family, friends and neighbours. Doctors, specialists and therapists, colleagues, clients and many more.

Many of you will know the impact you had, many others will not be aware of the vital contribution you made. I thank you all in making this book possible and the impact it can have to help others, who suffer, find relief and life beyond back pain.

Lightning Source UK Ltd.
Milton Keynes UK
UKOW06f1500190216

268728UK00001B/163/P